# pilates
## the complete
### body system

# pilates

the ## complete

## body system

## MICHAEL KING
### and Yolande Green

MITCHELL BEAZLEY

PILATES: THE COMPLETE BODY SYSTEM
by Michael King with Yolande Green

First published in Great Britain in 2003 by Mitchell Beazley,
an imprint of Octopus Publishing Group Limited,
2–4 Heron Quays, London E14 4JP

ISBN  1-84000-690-0

A CIP catalogue record for this book is available from the British Library.

While all reasonable care has been taken during the preparation of
this edition, neither the publisher, editors, nor the authors can accept
responsibility for any consequences arising from the use thereof or
from the information contained therein.

Executive Editor: Vivien Antwi
Executive Art Editor: Christine Keilty
Project Editor: Peter Taylor
Design: Peter Gerrish
Production: Alix McCulloch, Alexis Coogan
Copy-editor: Emma Clegg
Proofreader: Siobhan O'Connor
Indexer: Sandra Shotter
Photography: Ruth Jenkinson
Models: Nancy Markwick, Malcolm Muirhead


Set in Franklin Gothic and Walbaum


Printed and bound in China

# contents

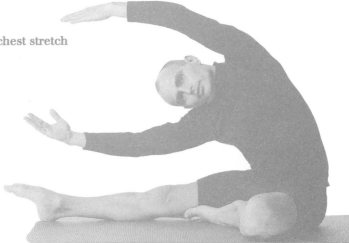

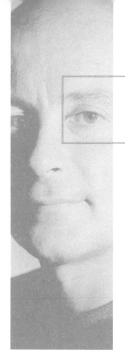

# introduction

Pilates is not a fitness fad; it is a holistic concept that will not only make you feel fitter and more flexible, but will also enrich your whole way of life. The series of movements will change how your body looks and give you a new physical poise and greater mental strength.

During my years as an exercise instructor, I have witnessed many fashionable shifts in the fitness industry – from high to low aerobics, from slide to step, and from spinning to core and functional training. Some of these changes have been introduced because of safety concerns over certain movements or ways of exercising. The advantage of a Pilates system, in contrast, is that the movements can be gentle on your body. The technique can also be effectively used to complement other exercise regimes.

I am one of a third generation of Pilates instructors following Joseph Pilates, and writing this book is part of my effort to give others an insight into the power of the Pilates way. I would like to pass on all the information and knowledge that I have developed over my years working in the fitness industry, training people in the physical skills that they can use to enrich the quality of their lives.

It is very exciting to witness the current popularity of Pilates. From the perspective of someone with a back injury who has worked with many different types of exercise, I have seen the value of the technique and the way that it changes people. You may believe that a hunched posture is part of growing older, but this is not the case. If we pay regular attention to our bodies and invest in them with stretching, challenging exercises, then we can benefit by feeling fitter and more attractive. We can also maintain these benefits as we become older.

## Pacing yourself

Undertaking advanced moves when you are at the beginning of a Pilates programme is the same as suggesting that a yoga novice start with an advanced yoga class. The original Pilates moves are advanced and inappropriate for those who are unfamiliar with the correct techniques. If you challenge yourself with Pilates exercises that are beyond your level or uncomfortable to practise, then you will inevitably demotivate yourself. This book offers a guide for beginners, but also provides different levels of exercise, with many positions offering an alternative modification. If you stay sensitively attuned to your body and challenge yourself gradually, then you can move towards your ultimate goals at an effective but safe pace.

## Balancing your body

Pilates is a system of exercise that, when regularly practised, will improve your flexibility and strength. The movements will have a noticeable impact on your body in terms of general well-being, youthfulness, and flexibility, but they will also help to heal any long- or short-term injuries. Even moderate regular daily activities may result in recurring aches or physical problems. Sitting at a desk all day, for example, unbalances your body, causing the hip flexors (the front of your thighs) and the upper back to form themselves into a rounded position. Pilates will help to release such tensions and ease your body back into a more natural balance. It also helps us to achieve leaner bodies and to feel more poised, less anxious, and stronger mentally. The moves shown here are structured with this in mind and are all based on the movements that Joseph Pilates taught himself.

## Challenge yourself

Remember: don't always follow the movements that you like or those that display your strengths because it tends to be the exercises that least appeal that will challenge you most. This is important to rebalance your body and to accustom it to positions that are more demanding. Aim also to exercise equally across the full range of movements, rather than concentrating on particular ones and specific muscle groups. Always listen to your body, both when exercising and once you have finished, and be sensitive to any vulnerable areas.

## A holistic approach

Pilates is not an exercise regime to be compartmentalized in your life. It is a thinking way of moving and involves making a serious

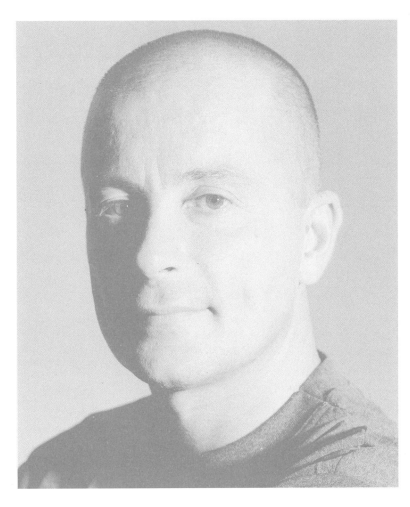

commitment to your body and your well-being. It will also be significantly more effective when combined with enough restful sleep, a healthy diet, and a regular complementary fitness programme. So Pilates shouldn't be the only exercise you do, but is an invaluable, solid support system for any other regular exercise that you are involved in. It is now accepted that the various fitness regimes – from aerobics or swimming to gym work and bodybuilding – are not inappropriate, but simply insufficient. While injuries are limited in exercise classes or gyms because of thorough warming-up

techniques and health-and-safety regulations, it is still common to pull muscles when lifting heavy items at home or work. This happens because an unbalanced exercise regime will not prepare the body for every eventuality. What we need to adopt, and what Pilates offers, is a way of training the different parts of the body to work together, to support each other and give your body the protection that it needs.

I hope that this book will pass on some of what I have learnt as a Pilates specialist and that the technique will enrich the quality of others' lives in the same way as it has my own.

# a history of Pilates

The Pilates system is the vision of Joseph Pilates. Born a sickly child, he resolved to improve his poor physical health and spent his life overcoming ailments including asthma, rheumatic fever, and rickets. He dedicated his whole life to becoming stronger and striving for physical perfection.

Joseph Humbertus Pilates was born near Düsseldorf in Germany in 1880. Rather than giving in to his various debilitating conditions, he resolved to build up his strength and overcome them. As he grew older, he took up many different sports, including skiing, diving, gymnastics, and bodybuilding. By the age of 14, at the end of the nineteenth century, Pilates was fit enough to pose for anatomical charts. Such dogged resolve was typical of his approach to life, and it informed all his future enterprises.

He maintained his developed system of exercise until he moved to England in 1912, where his excellent physical fitness enabled him to earn a living as both a boxer and a circus performer. When World War I broke out in 1914, he was interned on the Isle of Man because he was German. He spent his captivity nursing other inmates and training them in his own form of physical fitness.

During this period, there was an influenza epidemic, and while other camps suffered massive fatalities, the camp where Pilates was interned suffered none.

Pilates was then transferred to a hospital as a medical aid. This was when he starting using improvised fitness equipment with bed springs attached to the walls above the patients' beds. After the war, Pilates returned to Germany where he taught boxing and his new exercise programme to the newly formed German Army. Because he did not like what was happening in Germany, he then left for the United States in 1926.

When Pilates set up a studio in New York, there was a tremendous growth in interest in his technique. He took the dance world by storm, and it is said that every dancer in New York, including the Martha Graham Company, submitted to his spirited instruction. Apparently, when Pilates was teaching, he always wore a bathing suit, smoked cigars, and drank beer.

When Pilates died in 1967, he left no will and no successor to carry on his work. However, his wife, Clara, continued to run the New York Pilates Studio, and Romana Kryzanowska, a former student, became its director a few years later. Although there was no official school for Pilates teachers, Clara Pilates gave tuition to a number of aspiring teachers, one of whom was Ron Fletcher, a young dancer who had a chronic knee ailment through dancing. He went on to open his own studio in Los Angeles. A number of his other students did the same, and that is how the technique has been passed down.

Pilates was critical of the pressurized pace of life that he believed was responsible for people's mental and physical problems. This is why his ideas are still highly relevant today.

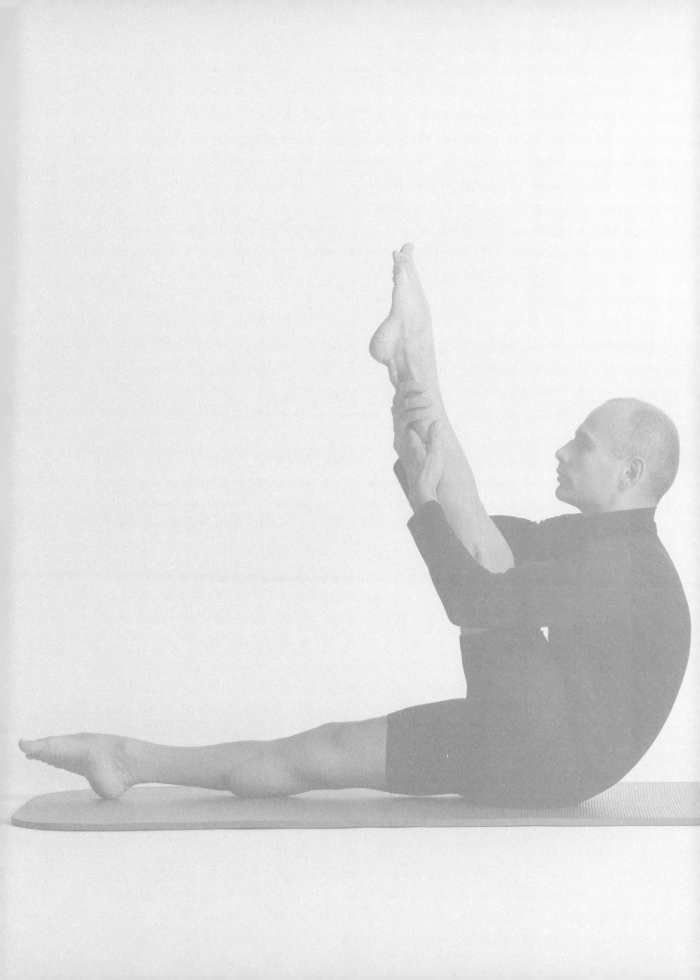

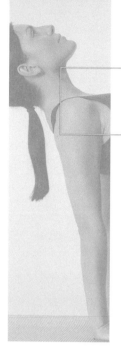

# why Pilates?

The Pilates movements stretch the muscles and pull them into a longer and leaner shape, rather than forcing them to tear and rebuild in a shorter and thicker shape as strength training does. It also gives a whole-body workout that challenges your body like no other exercise.

Pilates systematically exercises all the muscle groups in your body, challenging the weak areas as well as the strong. It balances the body, focuses on tight areas, and aims to increase strength and flexibility. When he conceived the original matwork exercises, Joseph Pilates was looking to stretch the body to the full to bring maximum benefit to the person exercising. Even experienced athletes may find some of his original moves difficult. This is because they use a level of muscle control and co-ordination that few of us are used to.

### All-round benefits

The Pilates system works the body as a whole and aims to co-ordinate the upper and lower muscle groups with the centre of the body. This has a dramatic effect on strength, flexibility, posture, and co-ordination. Whether you are interested in

Pilates for cosmetic, medical, or preventative reasons, the system of movements will strengthen your body and focus your mind.

### Anyone can do it

You do not have to be an athlete to be involved with Pilates. And while the exercises are designed to put a minimum of strain on the body, they also aim to challenge its capabilities. This means that anyone of any age and any level of fitness can do Pilates. Whether young or old, a fitness fanatic or someone who has never exercised before, you will reap the benefits.

### Offers achievable levels

Joseph Pilates' original book featured a series of 34 movements. Although I would like all of my students to be able to undertake the full range of these movements, as a responsible fitness leader I need to work around their capabilities. Joseph Pilates had an

exceptional level of physical conditioning that allowed him to use these moves, and such an advanced level has to be worked up to gradually. On a more moderate level, it is also highly inadvisable to try the crab or the leg-pull without easing your body into the movements first.

Pilates developed his technique from instinct, and although the basic principles always remained the same, when he worked with students he adapted the moves according to their different requirements. So an essential part of Pilates is knowing what you cannot do. The advantage is that the moves can be practised at different levels, from starter level to the highly advanced moves that Pilates himself developed.

### Basic equipment

You don't need any expensive equipment for Pilates exercises, and this means that you can follow

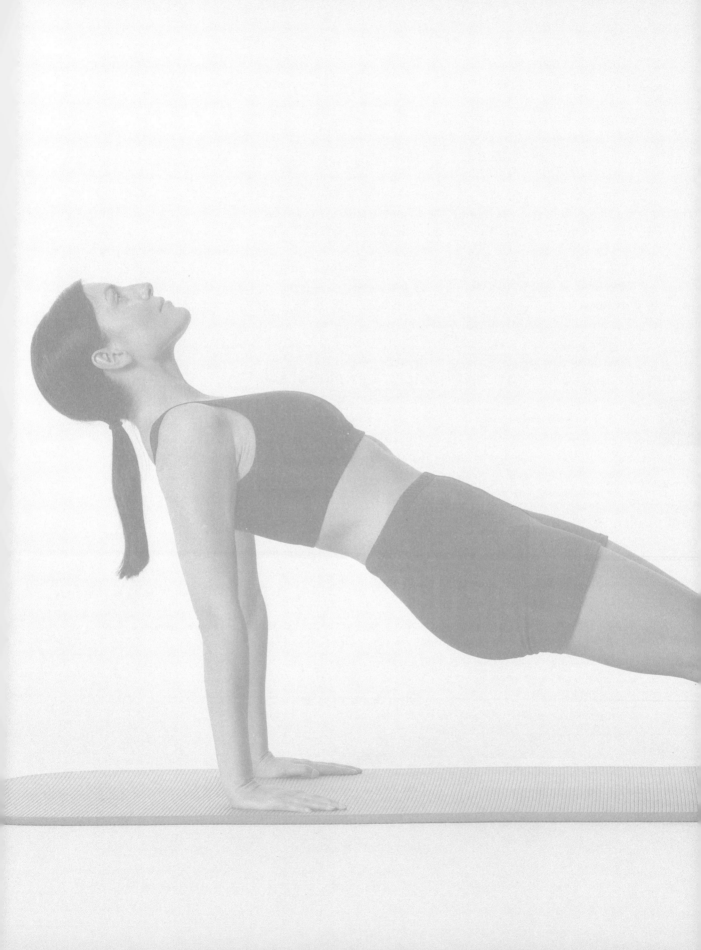

a programme at home with just a mat laid on the floor. The Pilates system is often linked to various innovative Pilates machines, equipment which can form an integral part of the exercises. However, remember that there is nothing that you can do on a machine that you can't do on the mat. Matwork gives Pilates a solid base, and what the equipment does is sometimes challenge the same movements with further resistance. Such machine work will accelerate the exercise and develop your skills to a more advanced level when you feel you are ready for this.

### Develops concentration

Known as the intelligent way of working out, this technique places a huge focus on concentration and discipline. Standard exercise regimes tend not to require mental discipline, but Pilates is different, healing and treating the mind and body on different levels. And because it works all the muscles in the body equally, simple everyday tasks such as shopping or moving furniture will also become easier and safer.

### Similarities with other techniques

Pilates and Yoga have certain goals in common, and most significantly they both advocate individual progress in a non-competitive format. The exercises also share an emphasis on stretching as well as the strengthening of muscles. Both Yoga and Pilates emphasize deep breathing and use smooth, long movements that encourage the muscles to relax and lengthen. Pilates is also similar to yoga because of the suppleness it brings. The difference is that while some yoga techniques involve moving from one static posture to the next without repetitions, Pilates flows through a series of movements that are more dynamic, systematic, and anatomically based. Pilates can also be linked with tai chi because of the considered quality of the movements.

### Popular support

Although Pilates has been around since the 1920s, an understanding of this programme of exercise that builds up your strength and your immune system has only become popular quite recently. Many Hollywood stars have endorsed the technique – among them Sharon Stone, Courteney Cox, Minnie Driver, Julia Roberts, and Madonna, who has even claimed that it is the only way to exercise. As a result, Pilates is no longer the domain of the rich and famous, and can be practised in most gyms and health clubs worldwide.

### Complete body system

Derived from the original Pilates movements, the physical programme that follows is designed around exercises that are achievable and safe for those who are new to the concept. Focusing on the most accessible level, it demonstrates the most vital part of the technique. Modifications are also offered within many of the exercises, and these enable you to vary the level of each one to suit you. The exercises will also challenge your abilities and offer you the classic pairing of strength and flexibility that is intrinsically linked to the Pilates philosophy.

### Ways of improving your health with Pilates

The Pilates technique is one that many people have adopted as a regular exercise regime to sustain them through their everyday lives. The following is a list of tangible ways in which the system can have a positive impact on your health.

*Pilates gives:*
- *Increased body tone*
- *A longer, leaner look*
- *No muscle bulk*
- *Improved balance*
- *More freedom of movement*
- *Heightened body awareness*
- *Reduced stress*
- *Increased energy*
- *Improved digestion*
- *A more effective absorption of oxygen*
- *Better circulation*
- *Enhanced immune system*
- *Increased strength, especially in the abdominal and back muscles*
- *Better co-ordination*
- *Improved muscle flexibility*
- *Improved posture*
- *Improved performance in sports*
- *A way of preventing injury*
- *An effective complement to other exercise regimes*
- *A general sense of well-being*
- *An improved sex life*

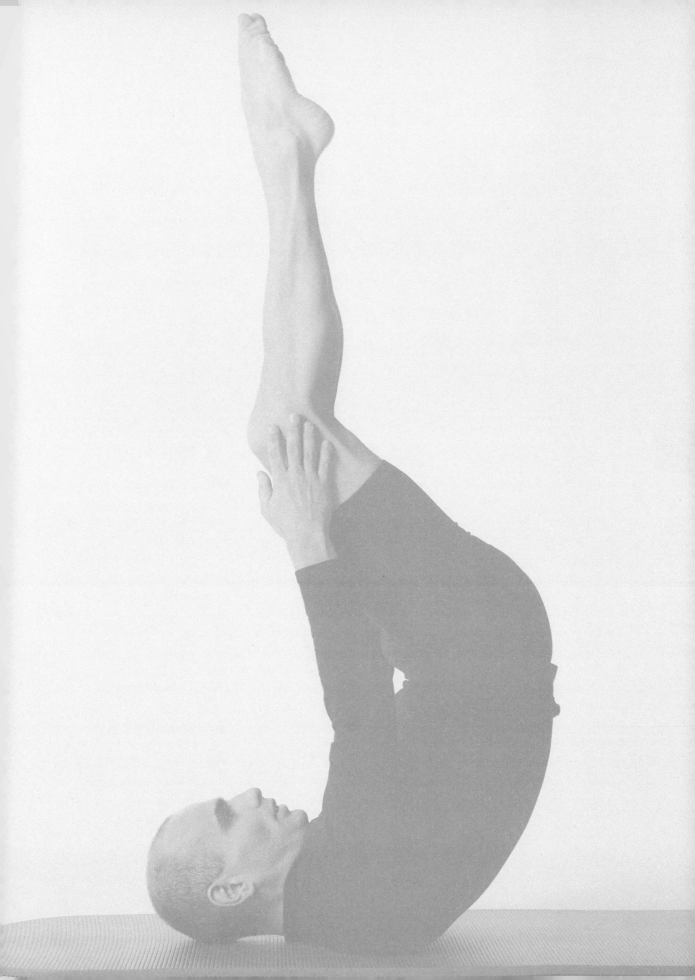

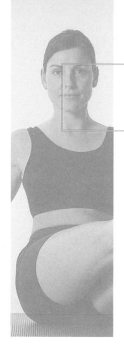

# setting your goals

What would you like to gain from this Pilates programme? You might want to look better, slim down, and define your body shape, or you may be more interested in becoming sensitively attuned to your body and using this to achieve a balanced, stress-free perspective in other areas of your life.

Those students who are new to Pilates will often cite their ultimate ambition as the achievement of a beautiful body, one that will attract others and increase confidence. When regularly followed, Pilates can help you to reach this goal. There are many other benefits too: some people start the programme in order to ease the pain of a back injury, build up their strength, or just feel better about themselves.

## A systematic approach

Understandably, if you are planning to change your body shape, it is natural to want to know how quickly such changes can be achieved. Instantly, is the answer. All you need to do is stand tall on your feet, pull your abdominals in, and drop your shoulders. Yet in order to maintain such a posture over time and for your body to change, a more realistic answer is three to six months of regular practise.

## Weight loss

One common goal that is not achievable by Pilates alone is weight loss. To lose weight, you need to work your body with your heart pumping at a high rate and to get slightly out of breath while exercising. The right heart rate for effective exercise and weight loss is 60–80 per cent of your maximum working heart rate. You should therefore do at least 50 minutes of cardiovascular exercise 3–5 times a week as well as Pilates.

It is also advisable to follow a healthy eating plan that includes plenty of fresh fruit, vegetables, proteins, and a restricted number of pastries or sweets.

## Focus on weak areas

You will need to understand where your physical strengths and weaknesses lie in order to focus on developing exercises that will challenge you. Weaknesses do not just signify a lack of muscular strength, but also relate to tight areas of your body that hold you back from fully performing a task: this might mean tight hamstrings, a tight back, or tension in the neck and shoulders. Remember that an inflexible body will result in the same problems as one with no muscular strength.

You will find that the exercises that you least enjoy are generally those that your body needs to spend more time on. In the same way, those that are easier will need to be practised less.

## Reshaping the body

A good posture and longer, leaner muscles will make you look and feel a new person. Work with the natural gifts of your body, whatever its characteristics, recognizing that you cannot replace it with a new one, but that you can make the best of the one you have. Pilates will help you on this journey.

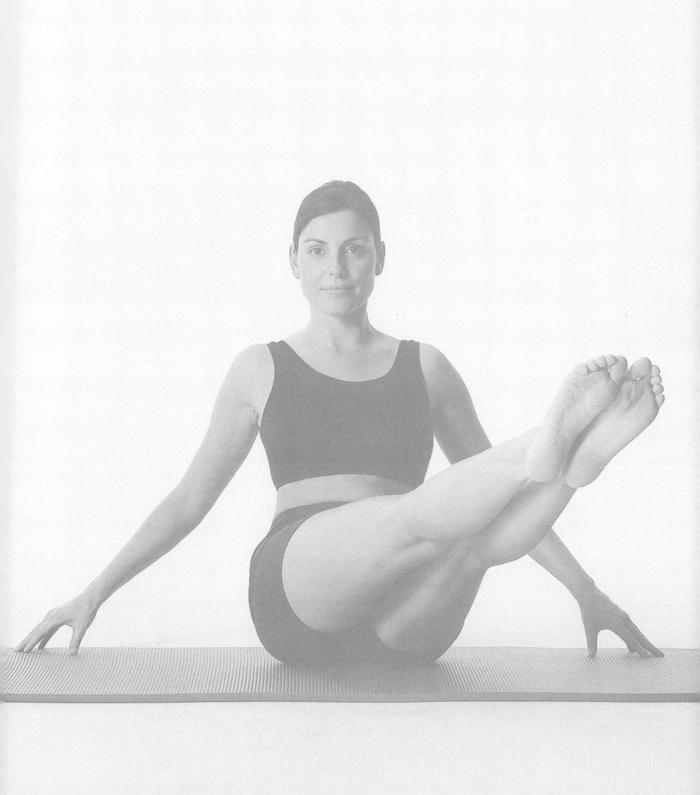

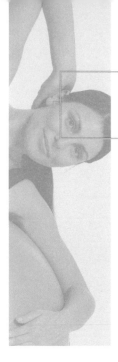

# preventing pain

We all have niggling pains that indicate tension in our body. We should never ignore these symptoms, but should use them to identify which areas need more strengthening or more stretching and mobility. Pilates trains the body to prevent injury and to maintain good posture and movement.

In order to have good posture, we also need to develop good muscle balance. Indeed, most injuries are related in some way to bad posture or muscular imbalances. These types of problems can occur for many reasons. Repetitive movements can be one cause, such as when a squash player continuously practises their swing on one side of the body. If they step and rotate in exactly the same pattern whenever they play squash, this will result in the shortening of one set of muscles and the lengthening and stretching of another.

Another way of unbalancing muscles is when people spend long periods of time driving or working at a desk. This means that the body is kept in a forward position with the shoulders generally forwards and lifted. This can be aggravated by repeated rotations to one side to answer the telephone, or having the receiver

tucked under your ear with your shoulder lifted as you continue to talk and work. These are just some examples: in fact, any repeated activity creates a habit, a way of instructing the muscles and joints to move. These patterns destabilize your body's natural balance and make it tense, in turn leading to weakness, tightness, and the resulting danger of injury.

It is even possible to injure yourself while doing quite simple activities, such as carrying a shopping basket or picking up your shoes. In such cases, the simple, everyday movement is the catalyst that makes the body buckle under the pressure it has been coping with.

**Back problems**
Back pain is one of the most common and persistent of physical complaints. Whatever the cause, and there are many causes, it will be noticeably improved by

regular Pilates exercise. This is because the technique strengthens the muscles that support and stabilize the core. However, always seek medical advice before starting a new exercise programme, particularly if you have existing back problems. You may even be recommended to start Pilates with a trained instructor who can advise you on any pain you are feeling. Learning more about your posture and practising neutral Pilates positions will also help to relieve the discomfort of any general back pain.

The key to maintaining a healthy back (as well as preventing general injury) is to improve your movement skills and your posture. Whenever you are standing, seated, or walking, remain focused on maintaining a good posture and avoiding slouching at all times (see also posture on page 28).

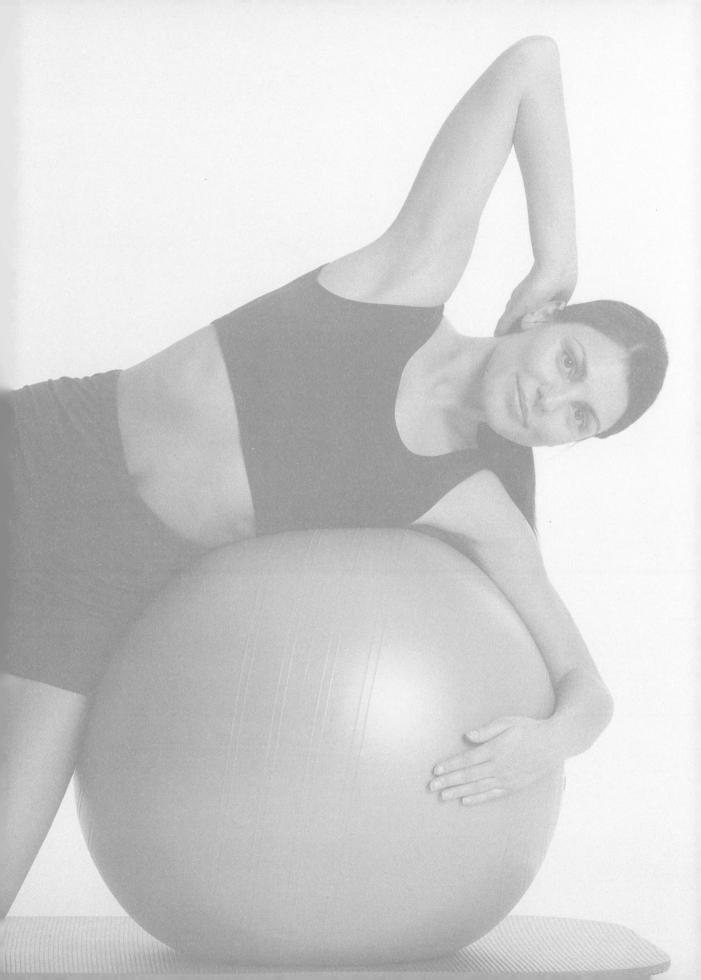

# principles

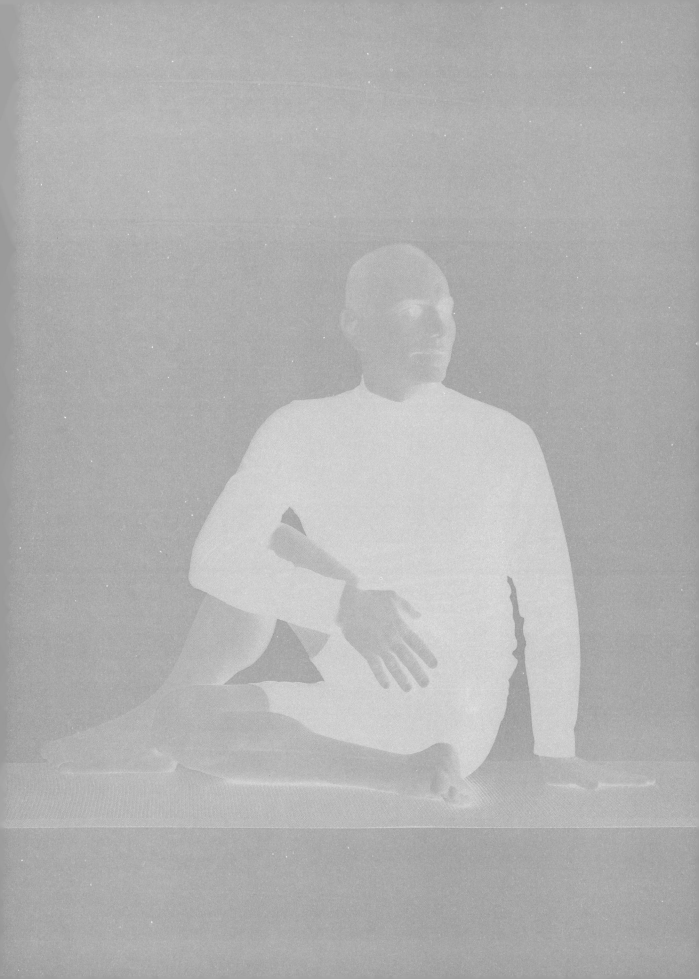

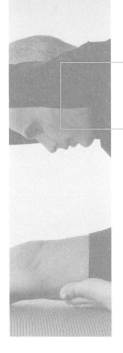

# concentration

Each Pilates exercise requires a thought process to control the movement. You also need to block out any other thoughts so as to fully focus on what you are doing. If you have practised yoga or martial arts, then this approach will be familiar, but for many this level of concentration can be highly challenging.

Good concentration skills are an essential part of the Pilates technique. Although other forms of exercise, such as swimming, aerobics, or gym workouts, can be practised by rote, a Pilates student requires mental focus in order to gain the most physical and mental rewards from the exercises.

### Making time for Pilates
Because concentration is linked to focusing on priorities, it is also needed when you are planning your exercises. Start with small sessions of 20–30 minutes, and aim to work up to an hour. It is better to have 20 minutes of a rewarding workout than an hour simply going through the motions of a routine.

### Setting the mood
There are a number of things that can be done to help you to concentrate. First of all, the place where you exercise should be warm and comfortable. Always switch off anything that will create any background noise before you start. Put "do not disturb" signs on the door, ban the children from your room, and divert any possible distractions that might interrupt your routine. Lighting candles and burning oil or incense may also help you to focus your mind.

Background music can be a successful addition to a Pilates session, but it has to fit in sensitively. Gentle music without vocals and without a strong beat tends to be most effective, as it allows you to move and breathe at your own pace. In contrast, classical music with sudden volume changes or heightened emotion can distract you from your mental focus. Even music that evokes a strong memory will break your concentration.

If you find it hard to maintain your concentration while you are exercising, try to clear your mind, listen to your breathing pattern for a few moments, then bring the mental focus back to your body.

### Reaping the rewards
You will soon feel the benefits of Pilates and your new ability to relax and concentrate will be particularly liberating. Good concentration will have a noticeable effect on your daily routine, enabling you to increase your mental focus and your clarity of thought in every situation and, most importantly, reduce your levels of stress.

The mind has a tendency to work overtime, and the hectic pace of the modern world makes it work much harder. This makes it even more important for us to have the skills to control our thoughts. Feeling tense will make you less able to concentrate, but mental focus comes with practice, and you will enjoy the resulting feelings of calmness and control.

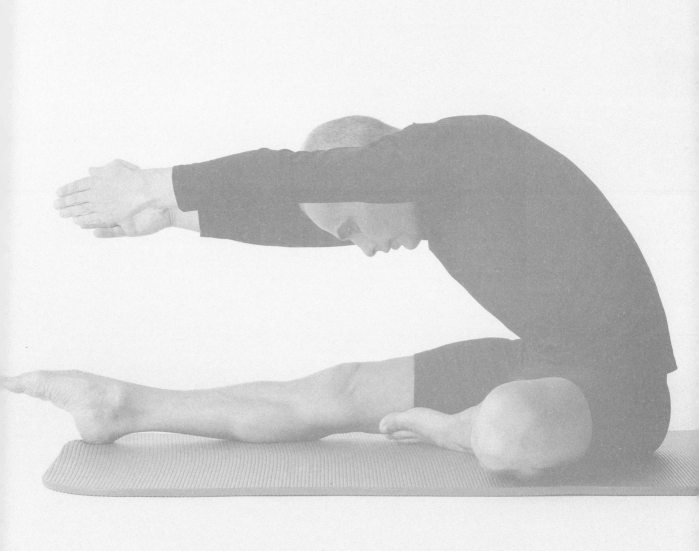

# breathing

Breathing plays a significant part in Pilates, and yet, for such a natural movement, it can be hard to perfect. The main principle for beginners is that you should breathe out when making the greatest effort using thoracic breathing, while also keeping the deep abdominal muscles slightly contracted.

There are many types of breathing techniques, and different types can make movements easier, harder, or more controlled. Correct breathing ensures a good flow of oxygen to the working muscles, which cleanses the bloodstream and energizes the whole body. It also improves concentration and aids smooth and fluid movement. As babies and young children, we breathe correctly, but as adults we tend to develop poor breathing patterns. A correct breathing technique can be mastered, but it will take time and patience.

**So how should we breathe?**
In Pilates, we follow a breath called thoracic or lateral breathing. This means breathing wide and full into your back and sides, opening the ribcage as you breathe. Think of your lungs as bellows, expanding and widening as you breathe in and closing down as you breathe out. This way of breathing works

the muscles between the ribs, called the intercostal muscles. When these muscles are working, the upper body is more mobile and fluid in its movements.

Pilates exercises are designed in combination with breathing techniques to work the correct muscles to create the required movement. The core muscles will always support this process.

**Muscles that make up the core**
The following groups of muscles make up our core or centre.
• *TA (transverse abdominal) muscles* are the corset-like muscles that wrap around the centre of our body.
• *Multifidus muscles* run down the length of the spine. They link two or three vertebrae and can create or block movement.
• *The pelvic floor* is the sling muscle that runs from the front of the pelvis to the power part of the spine.
• *The diaphragm* is the muscle

that lies under the ribcage and helps us to inhale and exhale.

**Thoracic breathing exercise**
Sit comfortably or stand tall. Place your hands on the front of your ribcage with your fingertips just touching (see picture opposite). As you breathe in, fill the lungs, open the ribcage, and let the fingers slide apart. As you breathe out, let them slide back to touch again. This can take considerable practice. To advance the exercise, move your hands further round so your hands are touching your armpits, and breathe to push your ribcage into your hands. If you can reach, extend your palms round to your back.

Another option is to place both hands on the front of the ribcage and breathe first into the right hand, then into the left hand, then into both hands equally. This will increase your body awareness and your breathing control.

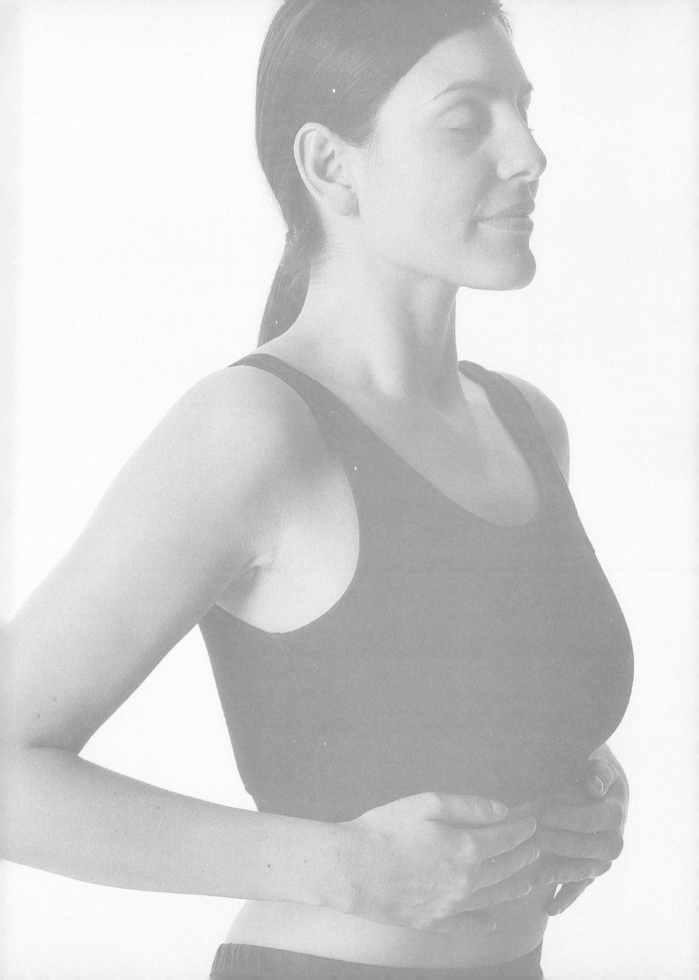

# centering

The body is designed to work as a complete unit. If you train to do this, you will have a solid centre to create the physical power for each movement. In order to visualize the body as an integrated unit, think of a conductor bringing together all the sections of an orchestra to perform a concerto.

In Joseph Pilates' time, there was no contemporary research to inform the development of his movement technique. What he advocated was established through personal experience and instinct. Current times, however, have seen a huge movement in the fitness industry towards functional exercise programmes, particularly in relation to torso exercise and core stability. This has meant that the centering principles of Pilates have become much more widely recognized and popular.

### The core

We have already referred to the core (see breathing on page 22) as consisting of four muscle groups, the TA muscles, the multifidus muscles (back muscles), the pelvic floor muscles, and the diaphragm. Your core strength can be imagined as a tree trunk, with the core being the solid supporting centre of your arms, legs, and head. If you imagine cutting through the trunk, the muscles of the body represent the rings of age in the tree. The global muscles are on the outside of the trunk with the rectus abdominus muscle. As you move in, there then follows the external oblique muscles, the internal oblique muscles, and finally the TA muscles.

### 30 per cent contraction

Every exercise is controlled or initiated from the contraction of the core muscles, either from the TA muscles or from the pelvic floor. This is because these two groups of muscles help to stabilize the body as we move.

For many years, Pilates practitioners would pull in the lower abdominal muscles harder as the movement became more challenging. Now, however, research has established that this is not the most effective way to work these muscles. Drawing in the abdominal muscles as hard as you can activates the core muscles with 100 per cent effort. This will tire the muscles quickly, and it will also not train them to operate effectively in everyday activities – when shopping or waiting for a bus, for example. Research has shown that the most effective way to train them is at 30 per cent of their maximum strength. This will allow them to be used throughout an hour's session without causing fatigue. They will also become naturally stronger and support you as you perform your daily activities. Work through the following exercises to help you to find your centre.

### Pelvic floor and TA muscles

Activate your centre either through the TA muscles (shown opposite) or by using the pelvic floor muscles. Research has shown that it is not productive to use both muscles together, so when following your routine, try to activate your centre by using just one group of muscles.

### Activating the TA muscles

Imagine that you have a belt around your waist and that the abdominal muscles draw in when you tighten it. Use this image to follow stages 1–3 below to establish the most efficient level at which to perform the exercises.

### Activating the pelvic floor

The pelvic floor runs from the front of the pelvis to the lower spine and supports you like a sling. This is one of the hardest muscles to activate, but when you master the movement, then it will be easy to practise wherever you are without anyone knowing.

Imagine your pelvic floor is the floor of an elevator. As you breathe out, draw up the elevator as far as you can to the tenth floor. Then release this halfway to the fifth floor and then a little further to the third floor. This is the level of exertion that you want to follow in the programme. Continue the exercise with the following pattern: move the lift to the tenth floor, return to the ground floor, up again to the fifth floor, and back to the ground floor. Finally go up to the third floor and back down.

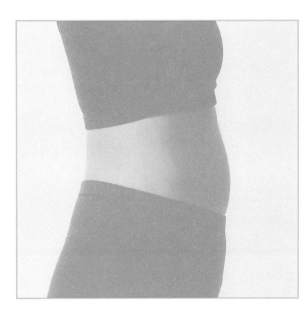

1 In a standing position, allow your abdominal muscles to relax and dome. Don't push them out, and instead become aware how the rest of your body feels as you release the muscles.

2 As you breathe out, draw in the abdominal muscles as far as you can. Imagine that a belt or corset is being tightened around you and that it will be tightened right up to the last notch. This is 100 per cent effort.

3 Relax the muscles halfway to reach the fifth notch on the belt. Think of this as 50 per cent effort. Then release them a little more to the third notch, or 30 per cent effort. This is the efficient level at which to work throughout your programme.

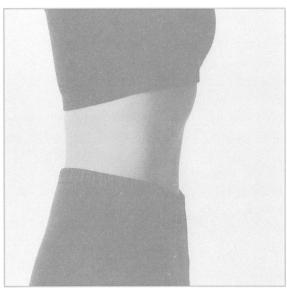

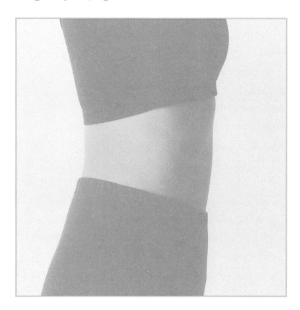

# control

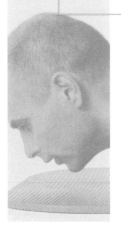

Good posture can be achieved only when the body is under perfect control. When doing the exercises, aim for slow, studied movements, and allow them to flow from start to finish to form a continuous sequence. Continue in this way until you have completed the total number of repetitions.

Working with the weight of your body against the natural pull of gravity requires considerable control. Yet we are all accustomed to controlling our bodies: the process of walking is not a haphazard series of movements, but a controlled sequence that we learn from childhood. However, many of us, quite unconsciously, develop bad habits in the way that we move that may later affect our physical health.

Maintaining control means ensuring that the body moves with purpose and direction at all times. A controlled movement involves making the relevant muscles and joints work to their full capacity while at the same time not wasting any energy. This concept is integral to the philosophy of Pilates.

Pilates exercises strengthen the body, and the slower, and more controlled, the movements, the greater the strength that we gain from them.

### Visualization
The use of visual associations can be enormously effective when working with Pilates. Visualization can help you to understand how to control your movements and also how to gain the most from your workouts. For example, we have already said that Pilates exercises need to be continuous and to flow from one stage to another quite freely, without interruption. So, if you are trying a new movement, it can be helpful to think at the same time of a Ferris wheel at a fairground – with the wheel turning slowly and deliberately. Or, instead, think of a tightrope walker at the circus. In order to stay on the rope, she has to maintain perfect control of her body and so has to move slowly and deliberately from one end of the rope to the other. Such visualizations are used throughout this book to give you a deeper insight into how each exercise should feel.

### The powerhouse
In disciplines such as tai chi, it is believed that the powerhouse is the store of the chi, or life energy. With physical movements, the energy is generated from the powerhouse, then carried to the relevant part of the body to give it power. This is equivalent to the core or centre in Pilates.

### Graceful control
When practising Pilates, make every movement as smooth and graceful as you can. To use a visualization, imagine that you are a dancer performing a movement on a stage in front of an audience, and you want to impress them with your grace and poise.

Think, too, about every part of your body as you move. Does each part have an important role in the execution of the movement, and are both sides of your body working at the same level? If not, rebalance yourself so that each part has an equal role.

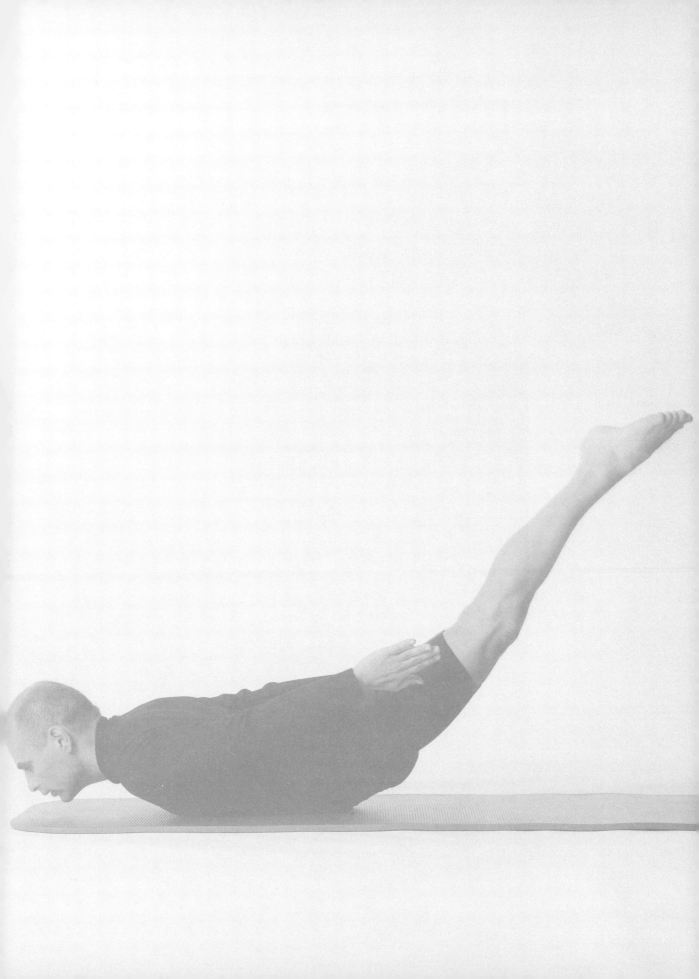

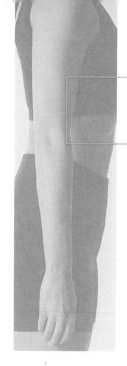

# posture

Good posture is vital. Having bad posture will prevent your body from functioning efficiently, and it will also undermine your balance and co-ordination. The danger is that if we develop a habit of having bad posture, our body will accept it as normal and will learn to suffer any associated aches and pains.

Poor posture can lead to many adverse symptoms, which include:
- *Fatigue*
- *Neck and shoulder tension*
- *Headaches*
- *Impaired balance and co-ordination*
- *Muscular weakness*
- *Poor circulation*
- *Tension and stress*
- *Digestive problems*
- *Aching and painful joints*

**Correcting poor posture**
There are the three main types of problematic posture: sway-back (see stage 1 opposite), lordosis (see stage 2 opposite), and kyphosis, although it is also possible to have a combination. Poor posture can be corrected, but it will take time and patience. As well as realignment exercises, you will need to give your body time to adjust to a different position. Some bad postures can be corrected surprisingly quickly, but others will need more time to remedy.

**Good posture**
An ideal posture will have all the joints in a neutral position, so that they are without stress and following the natural alignment of the bones. A neutral position will reduce wear on the joints, promote balance, and keep the muscles around the joints in correct alignment. This allows the internal organs to feel comfortable and to function efficiently. It is important that you establish a neutral position before you start each exercise.

**The plumbline test**
Assess your posture in front of a full-length mirror, wearing just your underwear. Stand side-on, and turn your head to the mirror.
   Imagine a plumbline hanging from your ear and look at the joints that the line runs through. With a healthy posture, the line should run through the ear lobe, the centre of the neck, the tip of the shoulder, the centre of the

ribcage, slightly behind the hip joint, the centre of the knee joint, and just in front of the anklebone.

**Typical characteristics of the sway-back posture:**
- *The head is forward or extended, so that the plumbline runs through the back of the neck.*
  - *The thoracic area of the spine (between the shoulder blades) is behind the plumbline.*
- *The abdominal muscles are short and weak.*
- *The pelvis is tilted backwards, but is slightly in front of the plumbline.*
- *The pelvis is positioned slightly further forwards than the feet.*
- *The curve of the lower spine is reduced and looks flat.*
- *The hip flexors are long and weak.*
- *The hamstrings are shortened.*
- *The gluteal muscles (in the bottom) look weak and flat, and are often without tone.*
- *The knees are locked back.*

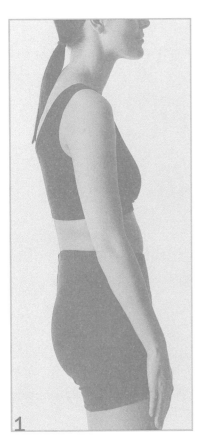

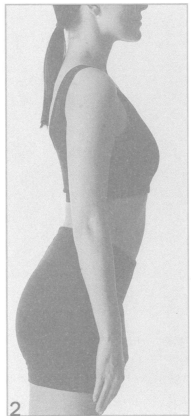

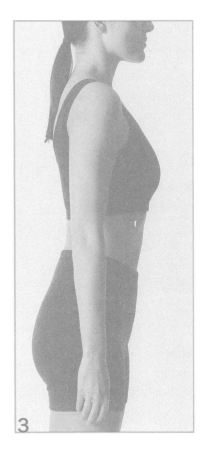

**1** Sway-back posture, often called the slouch position, is common amongst teenagers.

**2** The lordotic posture is characterized by an increased curve in the lower part of the spine.

**3** With an ideal posture, gravity is evenly distributed and all joints are in their neutral position.

**Suitable exercises for sway-back:**
*Rolling back, hamstring stretch, roll-up, swan dive, double-leg stretch, and push-up.*

**Typical characteristics of the lordotic posture:**
- *The head is in front of the plumbline.*
- *The thoracic area of the spine is behind the plumbline.*
- *The ribcage is flared and lifted.*
- *The pelvis is anteriorly rotated (tilted forwards).*
- *The position of the pelvis affects the curve of the lower spine and increases the size of the curve.*

- *The muscles of the lower spine are shortened and tight.*
- *The hip flexors are shortened.*
- *The abdominal muscles are weak.*
- *The hamstrings are weak.*
- *The quad muscles are shortened.*
- *The gluteals are weak.*
- *The knees are hyper-extended.*

**Suitable exercises for lordosis:**
*One-leg stretch, shoulder bridge, rolling back, hamstring stretch, roll-up, and seated spine stretch.*

**Typical characteristics of the ideal posture:**
- *The head is in the centre of the plumbline.*
- *The thoracic area is open.*
- *The muscles of the chest are opened.*
- *The muscles of the upper back are lengthened.*
- *The shoulder blades are dropped, sliding down the back in a "V" shape.*

**Suitable exercises to maintain an ideal posture**
*Use a balance of the strength and flexibility exercises in this book.*

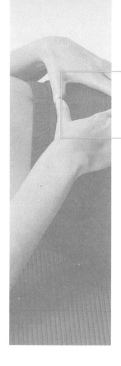

# neutral spine

A neutral spine is used to describe when your spine is in its most natural position. This will not necessarily be the position that feels most comfortable. It is quite likely that your "normal" posture has been created by poor habits and that you have just become accustomed to the way it feels.

Finding a position with a neutral spine can be a real challenge. It is essential, however, that you find your neutral position and sustain it before undertaking any of the Pilates moves. Once you have started on the exercises that follow, you will then need to learn to hold the neutral position as your body is moving.

### Training out of neutral

If your body loses the correct neutral position as you are exercising, then the benefit to you is lost. In this scenario, you are simply making your body stronger in your preferred, non-neutral position, one that has been created by bad habits. Training in a non-neutral position will also increase your chances of acquiring muscular imbalances, injuries, and increasing tension because your body is not adequately supported. It will want to revert to its bad habits, but you must keep easing it into neutral.

### Pelvis and spine

While it is important that all the joints are in neutral during the moves, this section focuses on the pelvis and spine. The position of the pelvis and the position of the lower spine will always affect each other. If your pelvis is rolled forwards, for example, the curve in your lower spine will be exaggerated, and it will therefore not form a neutral position.

### Finding neutral

You should always practise finding neutral before starting any exercises either by lying down or by standing – the principle is the same. Most people, however, find that lying down is always the easiest way to start. This is because the floor provides you with some support. Follow the stages that are described below.

### Stage one

This stage shows the spine out of neutral with an increased lower

spine curve. Start by lying on the floor in a relaxed position with your knees bent and your feet flat on the floor. Softly tilt the pelvis forwards so that the space under your lower back increases. Be careful not to push this position too far as it may cause you discomfort in your lower spine. See how each part of your body – particularly your legs, chest, and arms – feels in this position. Then relax back out of the position.

### Stage two

The second picture shows the spine out of neutral with no lower spine curve. In the same lying position, softly tilt your pelvis back and visualize imprinting your lower spine into the mat. Don't push this position too far, and stop if it feels uncomfortable. Notice how each part of your body – particularly your legs, abdominal muscles, back, and waist – feels in this position. Then relax back out of the position.

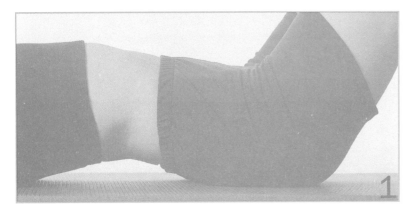

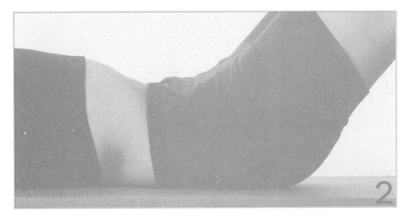

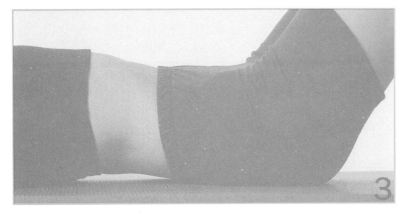

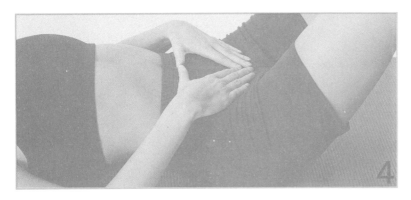

## Stage three

The third picture shows the spine in neutral. To find this position, shift your body between stages one and two, and find a position halfway between the two points. This should leave a small space under your lower back – imagine needing a space just big enough to slide your fingertips gently under the back. Notice how each part of your body feels in this position – there should be no tension in the legs, chest, or back.

## Stage four

The fourth stage shows the clock or compass technique, which is a way of helping you to find neutral. Often a more effective method, this shows you how to align your body from the pelvic bones (the hipbones).

Place your hands on your lower abdominal muscles, with your little fingers pointing down towards your pubic bone. Imagine that your hands are either a clockface (with the fingers pointing to 12 o'clock and your thumbs pointing to 6 o'clock) or a compass (with the fingers pointing north and your thumbs pointing south). Tilt the pelvis forwards and backwards, so that 12 o'clock or north is higher, then 6 o'clock or south is higher. Neutral is the position where 12 o'clock and north, and 6 o'clock and south are level.

Your body should be treated like a car: drivers check that the car is in neutral before they drive, in the same way that your body should find neutral before it exercises.

# routines

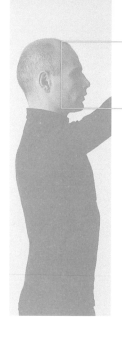

# warm-ups

The warm-up exercises are designed to mobilize, lengthen, and stretch the muscles in preparation for more demanding movements. Use them to familiarize yourself with how your body feels as it moves and to focus on your breathing and posture before moving on to the main exercises.

## the cat

Imagine that you are drawing up into yourself as you breathe out. Then, as you breathe in, gradually lengthen down and out of the position. Ensure that none of the positions is held and that every move flows smoothly into the following one.

| | |
|---|---|
| reps | 5–10 times |
| visual cue | a cat stretching |
| emphasis | mobility of the spine |

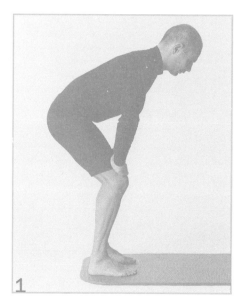

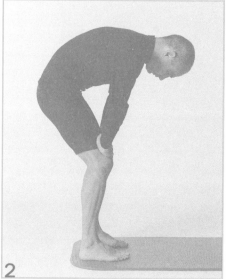

1 From a standing position, bend your knees and place your hands just above them without applying undue pressure on the knee joint. Your back should be flat and in the neutral position, and your head and neck should be in line. Try not to let your head drop or look up by concentrating on a spot on the floor in front of you. Breathe in to prepare for the next stage.

2 As you breathe out, draw up through the centre of your back in the same way as a cat when it is stretching. Open your back as much as possible without losing the shape of the lower body. As you breathe in, lower the back down to the neutral position. Repeat 5–10 times.

# swinging

The swinging movement should feel continuous and flowing. Only go as low as you feel comfortable with: as your body becomes warmer, you may be able to move down a little lower.

| | |
|---|---|
| reps | 5–10 times |
| visual cue | a rag doll |
| emphasis | strength |

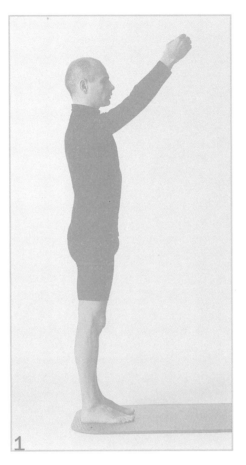

1 Stand tall in the neutral position. Then, with your eyes lifted, breathe in to prepare yourself and float your arms up in front of you without allowing your shoulders blades to lift.

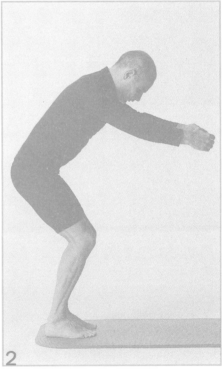

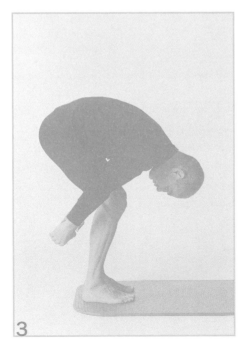

2 Softly bend your knees, allow your arms to relax, then slowly move into a great downwards scooping movement, breathing out as you go.

3 Continue with the movement while remembering to keep the knees soft. As you start to breathe in, slowly uncurl the movement until you are upright.

# standing spine twist

Concentrate on lengthening and maintaining the third notch on the belt (see page 25). As you rotate, focus on keeping your hips facing forwards with both feet planted on the ground, rather than allowing the hips to rotate with you.

| | |
|---|---|
| reps | 5–10 times each side |
| visual cue | corkscrew |
| emphasis | spine mobility |

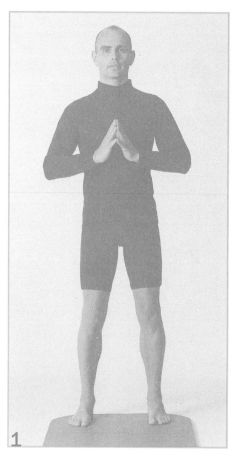

1 Standing tall in the neutral position, place the hands together in a praying gesture. Softly draw the shoulder blades back and then down into a soft "V". The thumbs should be placed on the sternum, the bone that runs through the centre of the chest. Keep the thumbs there throughout the exercise, because if they move off the sternum, the movement only involves the arms. Take a breath in to prepare yourself.

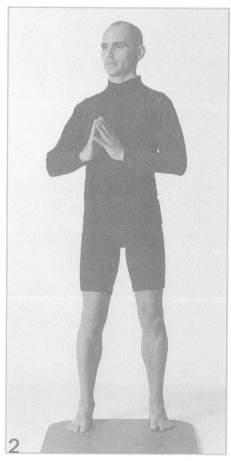

2 As you breathe out, slowly rotate to the right, keeping the thumbs on the sternum and the nose in line with the thumbs. Focus on making the movement come from the thoracic area of the spine (the area between the shoulder blades). The whole centre column should rotate as a single unit, so don't let the head or the arms rotate on their own. As you begin to breathe in, start to rotate back to the centre again. On the next outbreath, rotate to the left side, then back to the centre as you breathe in. When rotating, allow your breathing rate to control the speed of the movement. Try to lengthen a little bit further each time you rotate back to the centre.

# spine swing

Try not to overrotate the movement from the hips, and instead maintain your length in the lower spine. Keep the shoulders drawn down into the soft "V" and the belt muscle on the third notch (see page 25).

| | |
|---|---|
| reps | 5–10 times each side |
| visual cue | trailing hands |
| emphasis | spine |

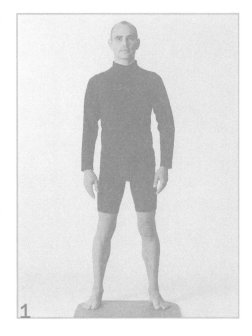

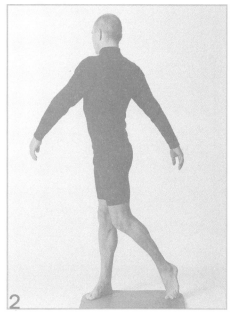

1 Stand tall with the spine in the neutral position and the feet slightly further apart than the hips. Breathe in to prepare yourself.

2 As you breathe out, slowly rotate to the right, allowing the left heel to lift slightly. Keep the arms relaxed beside you and your knees soft and relaxed. Allow your head to turn to look over your shoulder.

3 Breathe in and rotate to the other side, keeping the movement continuously flowing with no breaks in the middle. The arms are relaxed and the heels lift naturally as you rotate.

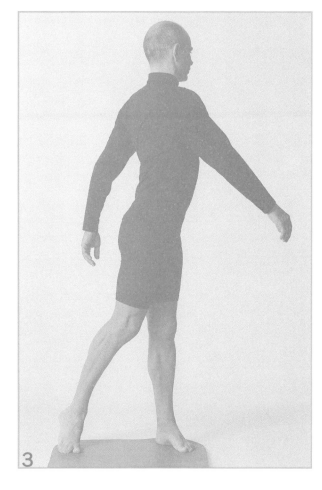

# balance 1

As you breathe out, slowly lift the leg. If you would like to challenge yourself, keep the leg lifted for 2–5 breaths before lowering it.

| | |
|---|---|
| reps | 5 times each side |
| visual cue | tightrope |
| emphasis | balance |

1 Stand tall in the neutral position, and keep your eyes focused on a point in front of you as if you are looking towards the horizon. Keep your hips as still as possible, and lengthen out your right toe in front of you, keeping the toe in contact with the floor. The hips should be still, shoulders drawn down into a soft "V", and the arms relaxed beside you. The belt muscle should be on the third notch (see page 25).

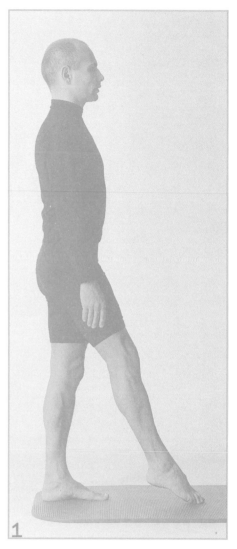

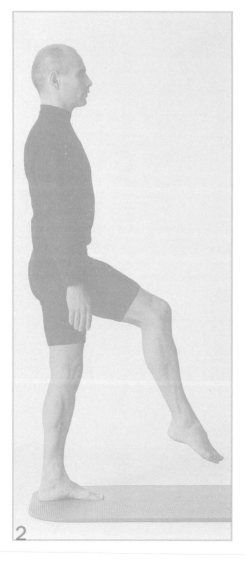

2 As you breathe out, slowly lift the right foot off the floor with the knee bent and the foot relaxed. Concentrate on keeping the left knee slightly bent, the hips still, and the weight even in the left foot. Imagine three points on the sole of your foot: one under the big toe, one under the little toe, and one under the heel. Aim to keep an even pressure across all three points.

# balance 2

Keep the weight evenly distributed across the left foot in the same way as the previous balance exercise. Ensure that the supporting knee remains soft.

| | |
|---|---|
| reps | 5 times each side |
| visual cue | arrow |
| emphasis | balance |

1 Starting from the neutral position, breathe out and lengthen the right leg and right arm. Don't lift the leg too high, and lean slightly forwards to allow the spine to remain lengthened and neutral. Keep the eyes looking down so that the neck stays in a neutral position.

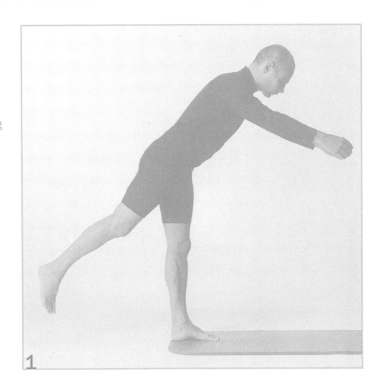

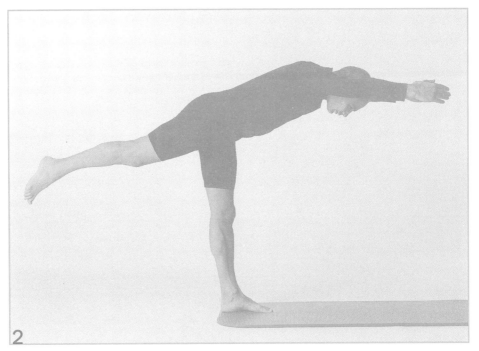

2 Keep lengthening through the movement until you reach a position where you feel you can maintain the balance and a neutral spine. Think about lengthening along the whole of the spine, from the head to the tail bone. As you breathe in, reverse the movement with control to finish in a tall, standing position.

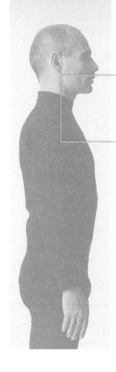
# essentials

These movements are the building blocks of the Pilates technique. Some of them have alternatives, depending on the level of intensity you require. An "advanced" move raises the intensity; a "modification" lowers it. Always listen to your body, and choose the level that suits you.

## push-up

Focus on this as a long, continuous single movement.

**! CAUTION**

**Soften or bend the knees if necessary: if your hamstrings or lower spine are tight, soften these areas more before you start.**

| | |
|---|---|
| reps | 5–10 times |
| visual cue | snail on wall |
| emphasis | strength in chest and triceps |

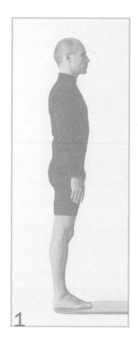

1 Stand tall in the neutral position with feet hip-width apart and shoulders drawn back and down. Imagine your eyes are looking over the horizon, and take a breath in to prepare for the movement.

2 As you breathe out, begin to roll your head and spine downwards, starting from the neck. Imagine each vertebra is in a chain that is moving link by link. Allow the weight of your arms to carry you forwards.

3 As you reach towards the floor, breathe in and bend your knees to enable your hands to touch the floor. As you breathe out, walk your hands along the floor. Keep your back level and think about keeping your bottom in line with your shoulders.

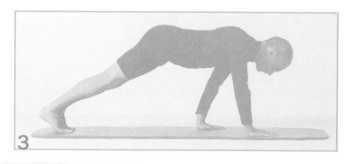

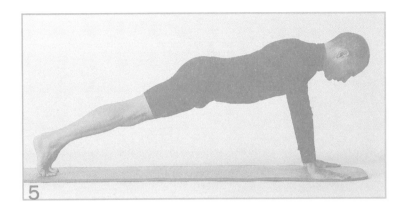

5

4 Before moving to the push-up phase of this movement, check that your body is in correct alignment so as to avoid straining your joints. Your hands should be directly under the shoulders, your shoulders drawn back and down away from the ears, your neck relaxed, and your eyes looking towards the floor.

5 Keeping the neutral alignment, breathe in and lower your body towards the floor. Draw the shoulders back and down as you perform the move, trying to keep the back in the neutral position and your bottom in line with your shoulders. Go as low as you can without losing the correct body alignment. Work back slowly through the positions until you come back to the standing position.

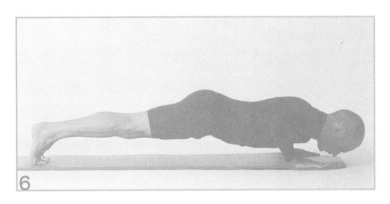

6

## modification

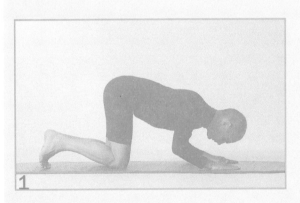

1

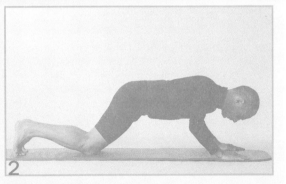

2

1 You can modify the push-up phase of the move by placing your knees on the floor. Once you have walked the hands forwards, slowly lower your knees onto the mat without causing any impact to your knee joints – this position is called the "box". The hands should be directly under the shoulder joints and the knees under the hips, with a box shape formed between hands and knees.

2 Once you have mastered the box position, then progress to a "long box", which adds more load to the upper body. Start in the box position and walk the hands away from the knees by about two paces. Realign the shoulders over the hands to create a slope from the hips to the knees. Keep this alignment as you perform the push-up, concentrating on keeping the hands and shoulders in line.

# swimming

Imagine that a laser beam is being projected underneath you, following the direction of your spine between your arms and legs. You must avoid touching the beam. Soften the elbows and keep the hips stable.

**! CAUTION**

**Avoid locking the elbows and having the knees too close or too wide apart.**

| reps | 20 times each side |
|---|---|
| visual cue | balancing glasses of water on back |
| emphasis | strength |

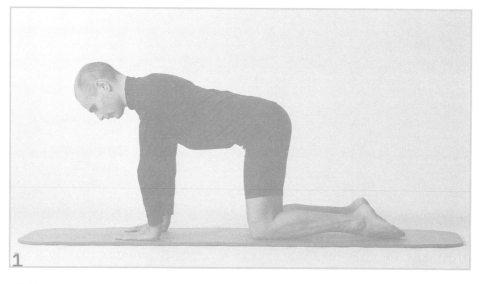

**1** Kneel on the floor, lean forwards, and place your hands under your shoulders. Your knees should be positioned below your hips, hip-width apart. Find your neutral spine position, keep your head level, and create a slight contraction of the centre (see page 30). Avoid rounding the shoulders, and keep your shoulder blades drawn down your back. The front of the chest should be kept open so that it does not collapse between the shoulder blades. This creates a strong base or starting position.

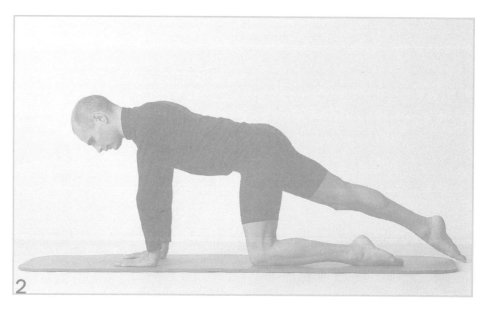

**2** Focus on holding this position while reaching out behind you with the big toe of your right leg as you breathe out, as if you were creating a straight groove in the sand behind you. Breathe in as you return to the starting position, placing the weight back on the knee. Now repeat the movement with the left leg. The challenge is to prevent the movement and leg transition from affecting the stable position of the body.

3 A different challenge, which takes some of the pressure off the wrists, is to start with the arms. In the same way as the leg exercise, reach out in front of you with alternate arms. Keep the fingers in contact with the floor, and control the shoulder blades so that they stay down and back. Make an effort to keep the upper body in the neutral position, and avoid taking all the weight on the knees. Imagine that your back is a tray with a full glass of water in each corner and that you cannot spill any water as you move.

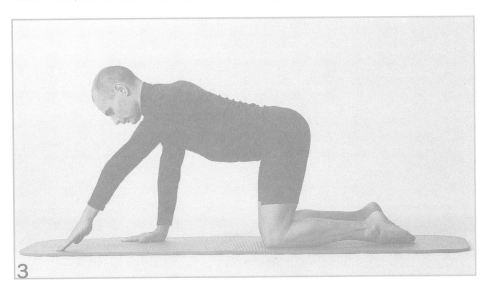

3

4 Once you have mastered this exercise, develop its range by using your arms or your legs. At full reach, raise the arm or leg that is off the floor to shoulder or hip height. Only continue with this movement if you are able to maintain the slight contraction of the centre. Finally, you have the option to introduce balancing skills to this exercise by lengthening the opposite arm and leg to create a diagonal across the body. Once again, the greatest challenge is on the transfer to the other side. Keep the arm and leg movement synchronized, lowering them before returning to the initial position.

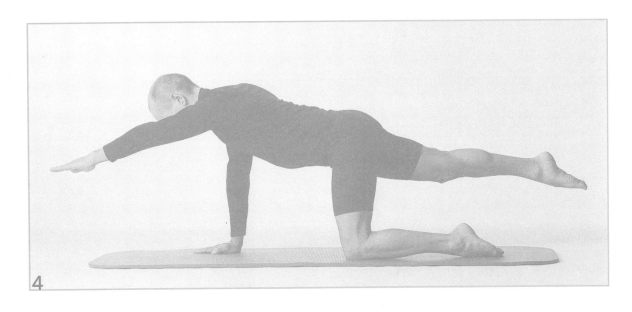

4

# plank

Imagine that your
back is a tray holding
a glass of water at
each corner: you have
to keep the tray level.

**! CAUTION**

**If you feel tightness
in your lower back,
tuck your bottom
under. If it still feels
tight, then drop it
down further.**

| | |
|---|---|
| reps | 3–5 times |
| visual cue | balancing |
| | glasses |
| emphasis | abdominal |
| | strength |

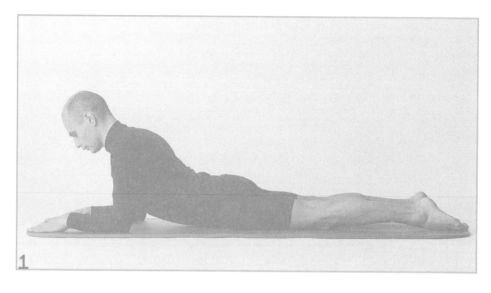

**1** Start the exercise by lying on your front
and supporting yourself on your elbows
with your arms lying parallel to each other.
Turn your palms towards each other, then
move them back so that your hands are
pressing softly into the floor with the elbows
under the shoulders.

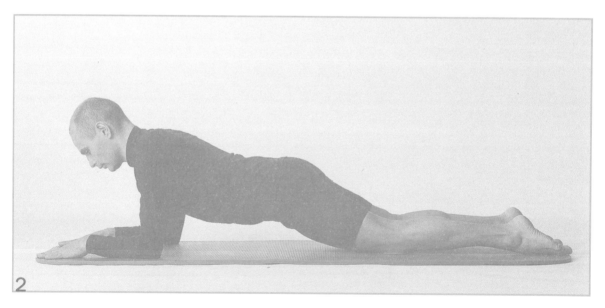

**2** As you breathe out, slowly raise your
hips off the floor, along with the lower
back of the ribcage and the lower abdominal
muscles, with your weight resting on the top
part of your knees. Keep the glute (buttock)
muscles relaxed. Draw your shoulder blades
back and down, and keep your spine in the
neutral position. If your lower spine dips or
feels tight, then relax the position down. Hold
the position for five breaths before slowly
lowering your body onto the mat without
losing control of your posture.

# plank into leg-pull prone

As you move your legs, focus on keeping your hips stable so that the glasses of water do not spill.

**! CAUTION**

**If you have tension in your shoulders, try adjusting the distance of your hands from your body in order to find the right position.**

| | |
|---|---|
| reps | 5–10 lifts each side |
| visual cue | balancing glasses |
| emphasis | abdominal strength |

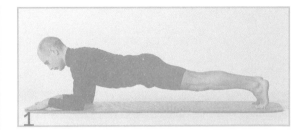

1 From the lying position, tuck your toes under, lengthen through your heels, and slowly lift your hips off the floor. Keeping the spine in neutral, float the knees away from the floor, and take a full breath in.

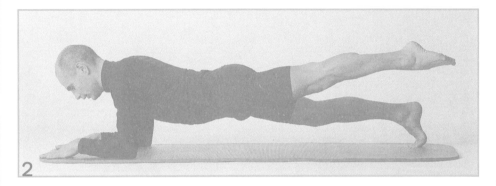

2 As you breathe out, brace yourself as you lengthen your right leg and lift it slowly. Keep your hips level and the balance central by imagining a spirit level lying flat across your hips. As you breathe in, lower the foot back to the floor. On the next breath, repeat the movement with the left leg. Focus on lengthening your leg behind you, rather than lifting it, and remember, if your lower back sinks or feels tight, then you should relax down.

## advanced

To challenge yourself further, try the advanced plank position with straight arms. Remember to maintain a horizontal back, paying attention to the lower part of the spine. If your back starts to dip or feel uncomfortable, then move out of the position and rest.

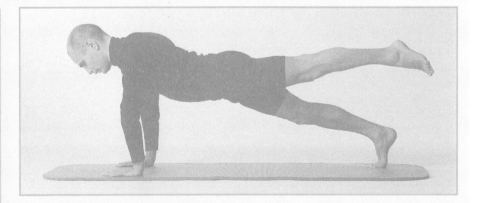

Align your hands directly under the shoulders, draw your shoulders back, and don't let your weight fall into them.

You should rather feel as if you are lifting the weight away from the shoulders. Hold for 5–10 breaths.

# side bend

Draw your shoulders back and down before you begin, and try to keep them there as you lift your body. Focus on lengthening your shoulders down and away from your neck, therefore avoiding sinking into the shoulder.

| | |
|---|---|
| reps | 5–10 times each side |
| visual cue | leaning tower |
| emphasis | waistline strength |

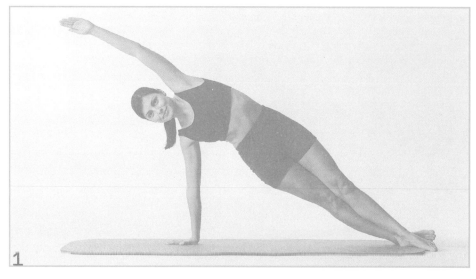

1

1 Sit on your right hip with your arm straight and your hand directly under your shoulder. Place your left leg over the right leg so that the left foot is just in front of the right. Breathe in to prepare, and as you breathe out, gently press the left foot on the floor and slowly float your hips away. Lifting your body as one unit, reach out and up towards the ceiling with your left hand. Breathe in as you lengthen at the top of the position. As you breathe out, slowly lower your body back down to the floor. Keep the movement constant, so that your hips softly touch the floor before then lifting up again. Your hips should remain one on top of the other, without the top hip rolling backwards or forwards, and your body should form a smooth diagonal line. Watch yourself in the mirror to make sure that your hips are not lifting too high.

## modification

Concentrate on drawing the shoulders back and down. Aim to lift the body as one unit rather than just lifting the hips, as this may take the spine out of neutral alignment. The move will feel slightly smaller than the main side bend.

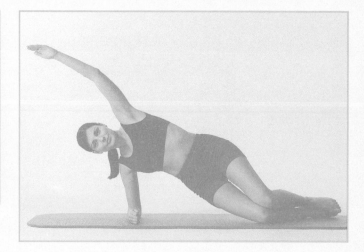

Rest your body on your elbow with the elbow directly under your shoulder. Bend both knees and stack the knees and feet on top of each other. Repeat 5–10 times.

# rolling back

The emphasis of this exercise is mobility, so imagine a rocking chair as a visual cue. Be gentle with your spine until you feel that the rolling movement becomes natural and you can return to a seated position with ease.

**! CAUTION**

**If you have a tight lower back and struggle to come back up from the roll, do not use the modification below.**

| | |
|---|---|
| reps | 5–10 times |
| visual cue | rocking chair |
| emphasis | spine |

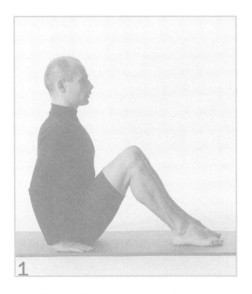

1 Sitting tall, extend upwards from your centre, imagining a taut string connecting the crown of your head to the ceiling. Bend your legs, and place your feet together flat on the floor. Place your hands beside you.

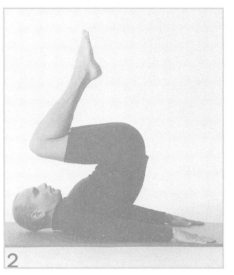

2 Take a slow breath in, curl your pelvis, and gently roll back as far as your shoulders. Roll back up, with your abdominals still contracted, and breathe out slowly. Complete the breath as you return to the seated position, and lengthen your spine to the ceiling. Aim to make the rolling movement as smooth as possible.

## advanced

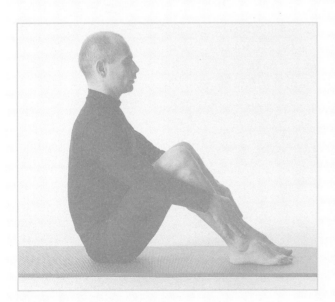

Once you have mastered the art of rolling, try it without the support of your arms. Sit in position and place your hands on your shins. As you roll back, keep your hands on your shins, and try to keep the distance between your chest and knees and heels and buttocks the same.

# swan dive

As you breathe in, lower your body back down to the floor. Allow the speed of your breath to control the speed of the movement, which should be continuous.

| reps | 5–10 times |
|------|-----------|
| visual cue | lying on thin ice |
| emphasis | spine mobility |

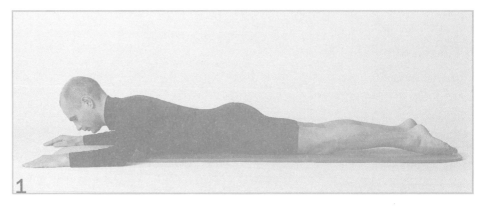

1

1 Lie on your front, and open your arms out on the floor, aligning your elbows with your shoulders. Make half a rectangle shape with your arms and draw your shoulders back and down. Keep your eyes looking down and your neck in line with your spine. Breathe in to prepare, and as you breathe out, float your chest away from the floor. The move should be small, so try not to focus on lifting the whole of the chest. Your elbows and hands should stay in contact with the floor: use them to push gently into the floor as you lift, but focus on lifting with the muscles in your back rather than those in your arms.

## advanced

Try to relax your glute muscles (buttocks). If you clench them, they will help to stabilize you as you lift, so the focus should rather come from your abdominals and back.

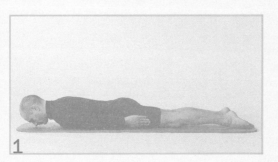

1

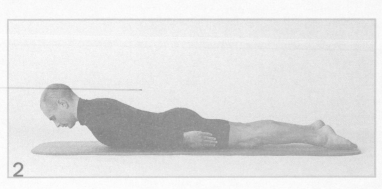

2

1 Starting from the lying position, place your arms by your sides with the palms touching your sides, and draw your shoulders back and down.

2 Breathing out slowly, float your chest away from the floor. As you breathe in, lower it again. Lift with the muscles of the back in the thoracic area. As you lift, lengthen the muscles in the lower part of the spine. If the muscles in the lower back are tightening or pinching, then relax down and rest, or return to the variation using your arms (above).

# advanced swan dive

This is an advanced move, so progress to this only when you have worked with the other exercises shown here for six months.

**! CAUTION**

**If you feel any discomfort in your lower back, stop and return to the other modifications.**

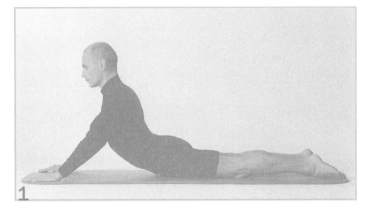

1 Lying on your front, extend your arms in front of you in the cobra position. Try not to compress the lower spine. Lift from the lower abdominals and hips instead. Breathe in to lift.

| reps | 5–10 times |
|---|---|
| visual cue | rocking horse |
| emphasis | spine and abdomen strength and mobility |

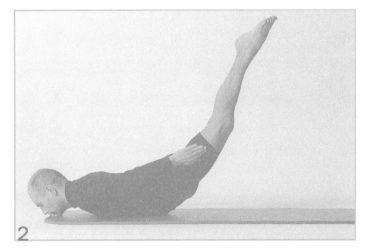

2 As you breathe out, allow your body weight to tip forwards onto your chest and your legs to lift behind you just like a counterbalance.

## modification with ball

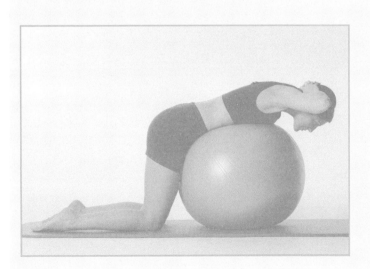

1 Kneel in front of a large ball, and curve your body over it. Place your hands behind your head with your elbows out wide and create a "tabletop" with your back and neck, not letting your head drop over the ball. As you breathe out, lengthen and lift your chest away from the ball, not allowing the ball to move underneath you. Remember that the movement should be small and controlled.

# roll-up

Imagine that your spine is a chain or a system of links: each area of the spine should work independently as you work through the movement to create a smooth, chain-like movement.

**! CAUTION**

**Keep your feet on the floor, and avoid spurts of speed as you roll up: the move should be smooth and continuous.**

| | |
|---|---|
| reps | 5–10 times |
| visual cue | the morning sun rising |
| emphasis | abdominal strength |

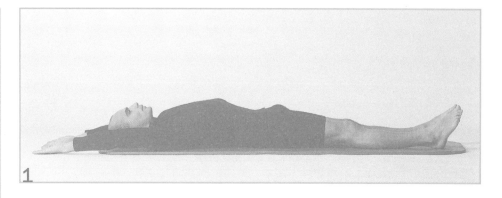

1

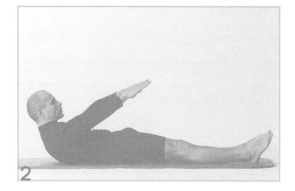

2

1 Lie on your back with your legs straight and your arms stretched over your head. Draw your shoulders back and down.

2 As you breathe out, begin to peel your head and shoulders off the floor, and slowly lift your arms towards the ceiling as you come up.

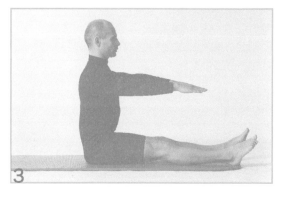

3

3 Continue to roll forwards slowly, peeling your spine off the floor vertebra by vertebra. Roll through the pelvis until you reach a sitting position.

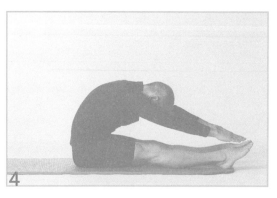

4

4 Breathe in as you lengthen out over your legs, stretching your arms towards your toes as far as you feel comfortable. As you breathe out, reverse the move and slowly lower your body back onto the mat: begin by rolling through the pelvis, then roll down vertebra by vertebra.

# leg-pull supine

It is important to keep your neck in line with your spine. To stop the head falling back, imagine that you are holding an orange under your chin.

| | |
|---|---|
| reps | 3–5 times |
| visual cue | Egyptian walk |
| emphasis | abdominal and back |

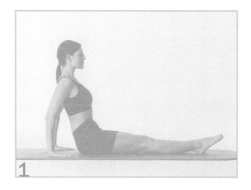

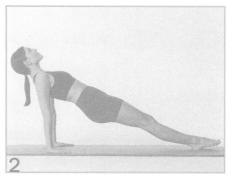

1 Start in a sitting position with your legs straight. Place your hands on the floor behind your bottom with your fingers pointing towards you. Keep your head lifted and your shoulders drawn back and down. Breathe in to prepare.

2 As you breathe out, raise your hips off the floor, keeping your legs straight and your shoulders drawn down. Don't lift your hips too high, and concentrate on lifting the body as one unit, creating a straight line running from shoulders to hips and toes. Hold for 5–10 breaths.

# teaser

Imagine that you are a concertina, folding and opening with each breath.

**! CAUTION**

**If you feel any discomfort in your lower back, stop immediately. Don't force the movement, but lift and lower to the point where you are challenged, but still in control of the movement and your posture.**

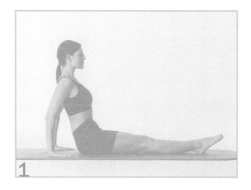

1 Sit tall with your hands on the floor close to your hips. Extend and raise your legs in front of you in a diagonal position. Draw your shoulders back and down.

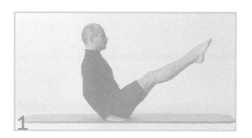

2 As you breathe out, take your hands away from the floor, and extend your arms out in front of you at shoulder height. Keep the shoulder blades drawn back and down, and hold the balance position. Lift and lengthen the body towards your toes, and breathe in at the top of the movement.

| | |
|---|---|
| reps | 5–10 times |
| visual cue | a slow horizontal dive |
| emphasis | abdominal strength |

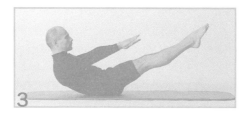

3 As you breathe out, lower your back down slowly, rolling through the pelvis until you find the point at which you are challenged, but can still retain control. Your abdominal muscles should be doming, or pushing out.

# the hundred

As you move your legs, brace your centre to keep a firm support. Keep both hips level as you lift your leg.

**! CAUTION**

**Remain focused on keeping your body in the neutral position. Check that the size of the arch in your lower back has not increased or decreased as you lift and lower your leg.**

| | |
|---|---|
| reps | 2 sets on each leg |
| visual cue | steep slope |
| emphasis | abdominal strength |

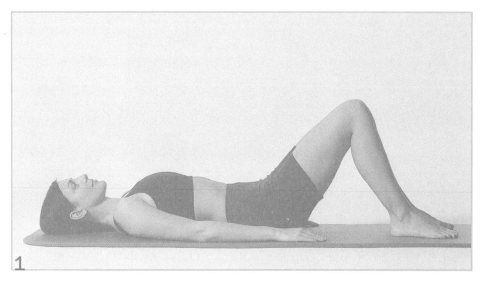

1 Lie on your back with your knees bent and your feet flat on the floor, comfortably close to your bottom. Find the neutral position, and with your arms by your side, draw the shoulders back and down.

Imagine that there is an orange between your chin and chest, and try to lengthen through the back of the neck.

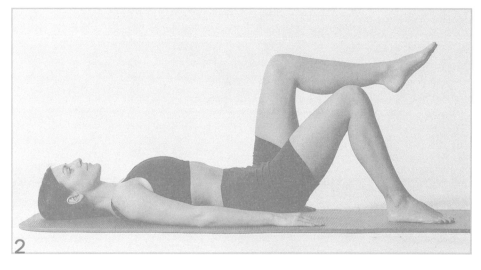

2 As you breathe out, lift the right leg to form a right angle, checking that the knee comes directly above the hip and that the foot is in line with the knee. Hold the leg in this position for five whole breaths. Concentrate on keeping your hips still and braced. On the fifth outbreath, slowly lower

the leg back to the starting position, bracing the hips to reduce any movement. On the next outbreath, lift the left leg and repeat the movement, again holding the position for five breaths. The goal is for the back to stay in neutral – don't pull up past the third notch.

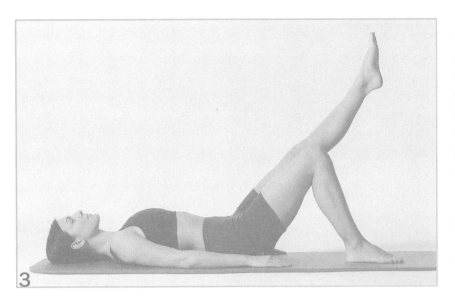

3 To challenge yourself further, lift your leg off the floor while at the same time lengthening it. Because the weight of the leg has been increased, you will need to focus on maintaining your neutral position. If you lose the position, lower the level.

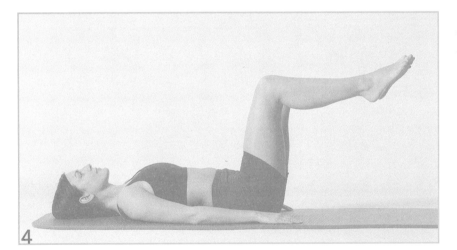

4 Once you have spent time working with the above levels, you can also try the hundred with both legs lifted. Lift one leg as shown in stage 2, and imprint your lower spine firmly into the mat. Then lift the second leg, and allow the spine to return to the neutral position. Hold for five breaths, focusing on not letting the abdominal muscles dome or the lower spine come out of the neutral position. On the last breath, lower one leg at a time, and return to the starting position.

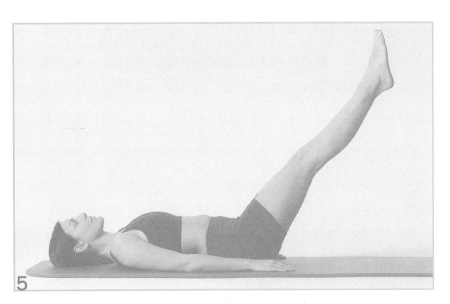

5 Once you have become confident with stage 4, push your muscles further by lengthening your legs diagonally towards the ceiling. If at any time you feel you are losing your neutral position, either bend the legs or lower them to the floor one at a time.

# shoulder bridge

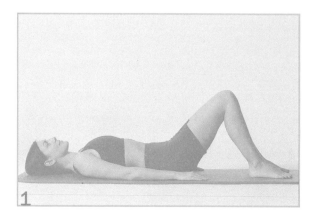

Keep your arms beside you on the floor throughout this exercise. You may use them to imprint the spine into the floor to help you stabilize, but avoid gripping the surface of the floor with your arms, therefore building tension in the shoulders.

| reps | 5–10 times |
| --- | --- |
| visual cue | ski slope |
| emphasis | spine mobility |

**1** Lie on your back with your knees bent, your feet flat, and hips and feet hip-width apart. As you breathe out, tilt your pelvis under and imprint your lower spine on the mat. Breathe in, and as you breathe out, reverse the movement so that you roll the pelvis back into neutral. Repeat 3–5 times.

**2** With your spine flat, slowly tilt the pelvis off the floor. Begin with the lower vertebrae one by one, and keeping the movement smooth, continue to lift through the lower spine, the middle spine, and up to the shoulder blades. Your hips and shoulders should create a ski-slope position. Breathe in at the top of the movement, and as you breathe out, slowly lower the spine back to the mat.

**3** To introduce arm movements, keep your arms by your side, breathe out, and lift into the shoulder bridge position. As you breathe in, float your arms up and over your head, although you may find that they will not touch the floor at first. Slowly lower the spine back to the floor as you breathe out. As the pelvis returns to neutral, breathe in and return the arms to your sides.

**4** An advanced option is to add the leg and balance movement. Keeping your arms by your sides, slowly peel the spine up to the shoulder bridge position. Brace your hips, and on your next outbreath, unfold your right leg and lengthen it to the ceiling. Breathe in as you lower the leg to restabilize and breathe out to lower the spine back down to the floor. Repeat with the left leg.

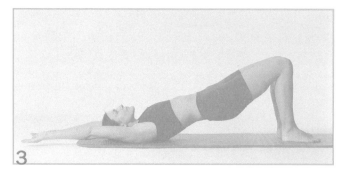

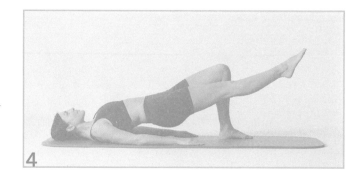

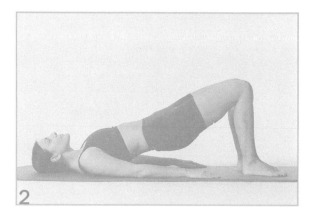

abs & back

**54**

ESSENTIALS

# one-leg circle

The main movement is the circling of the knee, but try also to focus on the top of the thigh circling within the hip joint as if it were drawing a smooth circle inside the joint. Don't let the weight of the leg drop heavily into the hip joint, and try to keep the hips level and in the neutral position.

| | |
|---|---|
| reps | 5–10 circles each way |
| visual cue | clock |
| emphasis | leg mobility and strength |

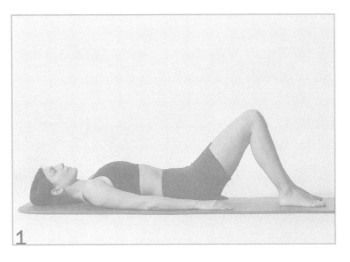

1 Lie on your back, with knees bent and feet flat on the floor comfortably close to your bottom. Find neutral, and with your arms by your side, draw the shoulders back and down. Imagine an orange between your chin and chest, and lengthen through the back of the neck.

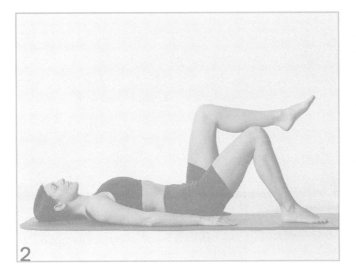

2 As you breathe out, lift the left leg to form a right angle: the knee should be directly above the hip, and the foot should be in line with the knee. Hold the leg in this position for five whole breaths. Focus on keeping the hips still and braced.

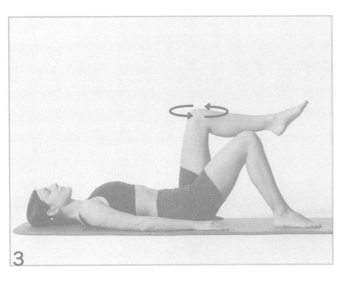

3 Keeping the left knee bent, draw a small circle on the ceiling with the knee, ensuring that it remains directly above the hips. As the knee comes in towards the centre of the body, breathe in; as the knee travels away from the body, breathe out. Perform five circles in each direction, trying to increase the size of the circle very slightly with each one. Once you have drawn five circles in each direction, breathe out and slowly lower the leg to the starting position. Repeat with the other leg.

# scissors

This is a strength movement and a development of the hundred. It will also tone your legs as you move through the various levels.

**! CAUTION**

**Only work to a level where you can maintain neutral without straining the back or creating tension in the neck.**

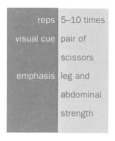

| reps | 5–10 times |
| visual cue | pair of scissors |
| emphasis | leg and abdominal strength |

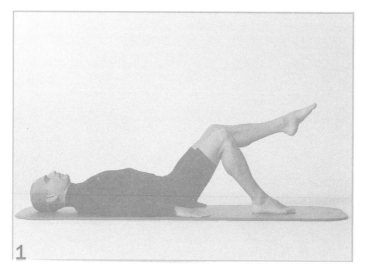

**1** Lie on your back and raise your leg in the same way as stage 2 of the hundred (see page 52). Lower the raised foot towards the floor as you breathe out, and raise it again as you breathe in. Focus on keeping your hips and your floor leg stable.

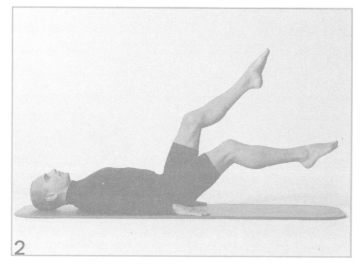

**2** Raise one leg to the right-angle position, imprint the spine on the floor, and raise the other leg to join the first. Return to neutral, and start to repeat the leg action, but as the first leg returns, take the second leg down. This sequence creates a scissor-like movement.

**3** The most advanced level of the scissor movement works the shoulders and legs, as well as the lower back and the abdominals. Straighten your legs and point your toes to achieve your full length. Raise one leg at a 45-degree angle to the floor, and set the scissor action in motion. As you adapt to the movement, the closer the leg can go to the floor and the higher the opposite leg can reach. Draw the shoulders down, and touch the thigh of the raised leg with your hands.

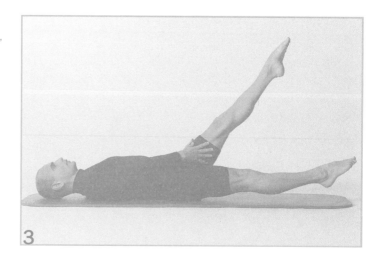

# one-leg stretch

Focus on stabilizing the hips and maintaining neutral as you lengthen the leg away. Your shoulders should remain drawn back and down.

**! CAUTION**

**Make sure that the arch in the lower back does not increase or decrease as you lift and lower the legs.**

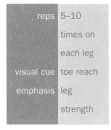

| reps | 5–10 times on each leg |
|------|------------------------|
| visual cue | toe reach |
| emphasis | leg strength |

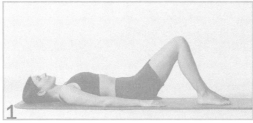

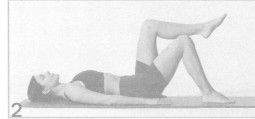

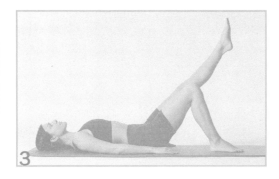

**1** Lie on your back with your knees bent and your feet flat on the floor comfortably close to your bottom. Find neutral, and with your arms by your sides, draw the shoulders back and down. Imagine an orange between your chin and chest, and try to lengthen through the back of the neck.

**2** As you breathe out, lift the left leg to a right angle. Check that the knee is directly above the hip and that the foot is in line with the knee. As you hold this position, focus on keeping the hips still and braced. Breathe in.

**3** As you breathe out, again lengthen the left diagonal towards the ceiling. Concentrate on maintaining neutral and keeping the hips braced. As you breathe in, return the leg to a right-angle position. Lengthen the leg five times, and slowly lower it back to the starting position. Repeat with the right leg.

## advanced

Keep your arms relaxed beside you: while they can offer you some support, avoid gripping the floor with them.

**! CAUTION**

**If you feel any discomfort in your lower back, stop immediately or take the leg up to a higher position.**

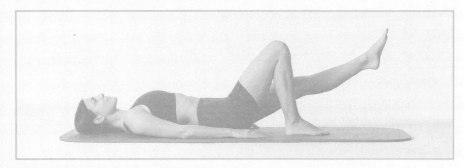

Once you have mastered the above levels, push yourself further with this modification of the one-leg stretch. As you lengthen the leg, lower it towards the floor: the lower the leg, the greater the challenge is to maintain the neutral position. Repeat five times on each leg.

# double-leg stretch

Focus on maintaining neutral as you circle the arms. The hips should feel braced, the shoulders drawn back and down, and the back of the ribcage should remain softly imprinted into the mat. If you do feel your spine lifting away from the mat, then combat this by reducing the size of the circles.

| reps | 5–10 times |
|---|---|
| visual cue | morning stretch |
| emphasis | abdominal strength |

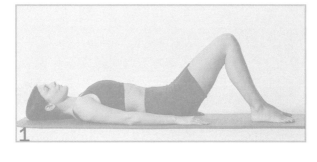

**1** Lie on your back with your knees bent and your feet flat on the floor comfortably close to your bottom. Find neutral, and with your arms by your sides draw the shoulders back and down. Imagine an orange between your chin and chest, and try to lengthen through the back of the neck.

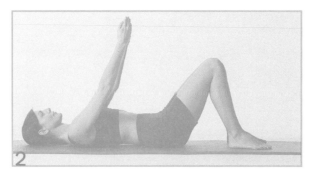

**2** Breathe in as you slowly float both arms up towards the ceiling. Focus on drawing the shoulder blades back and down.

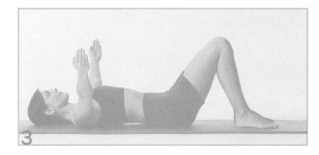

**3** As you breathe out, continue the circle round as if drawing two semi-circles on each side of your body. Start with small circles, and avoid going too near the floor to begin with. Focus on keeping the ribcage in neutral and the back of the ribcage in contact with the floor.

## advanced

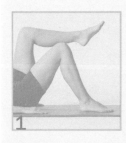

**1** Once you have mastered the arm circles, extend the exercise by lifting one leg as shown in the hundred (see page 52). Keep the leg lifted at a right angle as you circle the arms five times. On the last outbreath, slowly lower the leg to the starting position, breathe in, then repeat with the other leg.

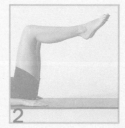

**2** The final challenge in this exercise is to raise both legs in the same way as stage 4 of the hundred and circle the arms 5–10 times. If you have not mastered the hundred, then work with just one leg lifted and one foot on the floor. Remember to imprint your back on the floor before you lift the second leg.

# seated spine stretch

Think of the movement as a single, long, slow sequence. Be careful not to strain your back, and try to keep all your joints in neutral alignment.

| | |
|---|---|
| reps | 5–10 times |
| visual cue | leaning over ball |
| emphasis | mobility |

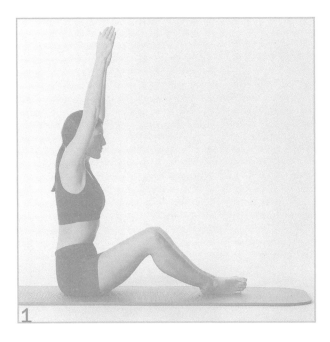

1

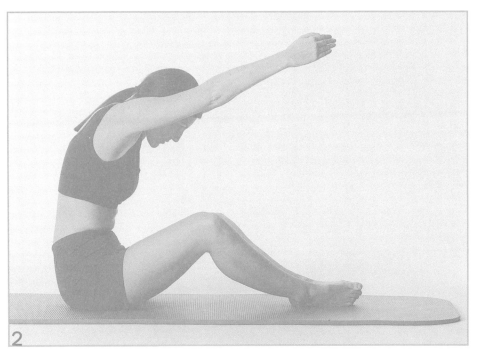

2

1 Sit tall in a neutral position with your feet hip-width apart and your knees relaxed. Raise your arms so that they are pointing straight above your head. Breathe in. As you breathe out, draw in the lower abdominals towards the spine.

2 Slowly start to bend forwards, rolling the spine down as you do so. Lead this movement with your head, let the chin drop to the chest, then allow the shoulders to roll over and the weight of the arms to carry you down as far as possible without losing control. Relax and gently bend the knees as you curl down to the floor. Pay attention to your hips, and if you feel that they are pushing out behind you, bend your knees a bit more, and don't go so low. You should feel as if you are folding into yourself.

# the can can

Focus on keeping the spine in neutral. The movement should come from the pelvis rather than from the lower spine.

**! CAUTION**

**If you feel any discomfort in the lower back, use the modification instead. The position of the hands is only for additional support.**

| | |
|---|---|
| reps | 5–10 full |
| | sets |
| visual cue | can can |
| emphasis | leg |
| | strength |

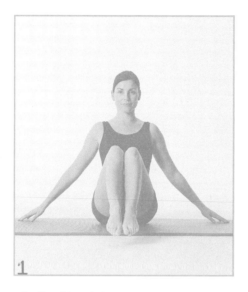

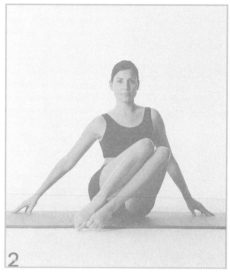

**1** Sit tall in a balanced position with your feet comfortably close to your bottom. Your hands should be out to the sides in a balancing position, and feet and hands should only lightly touch the floor.

**2** As you breathe out, rotate your hips to the left. The hands can be used to stabilize the position, but do not let the arms support too much weight. Breathe in as your knees come back to the centre.

**3** Keeping the knees together, tuck the right leg underneath towards the bottom. Focus on sitting tall and balancing while bracing your centre. Slowly lengthen the top leg as you breathe out, bend the knees, and repeat to the other side.

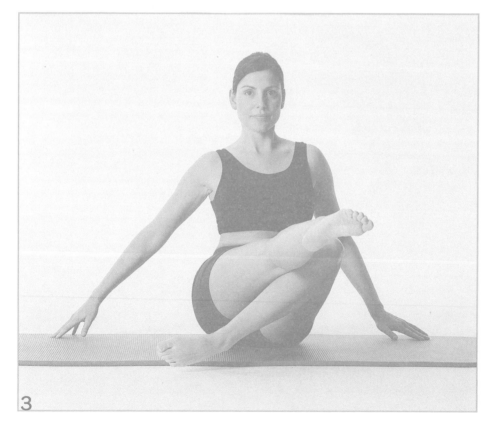

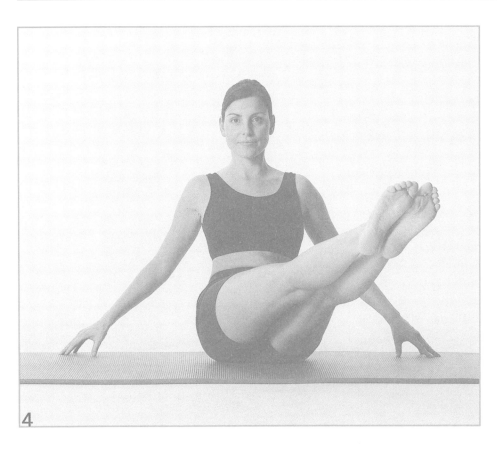

4 This is the most advanced move. As you breathe out, lengthen both legs back out to the left side. As you breathe in, bend the knees and rotate back to the centre. Repeat on the other side.

## modification

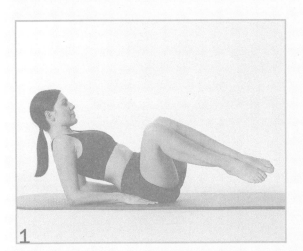

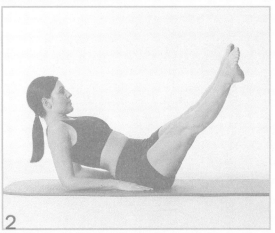

1 To add more stability, lay back on your elbows, bend the legs close to the bottom, and draw the shoulders back and down, keeping the centre braced.

2 As you breathe out, rotate to the right, and lengthen the legs as before.

# hip circles

Aim to keep the spine in neutral while doing this movement. Also try to keep the distance equal between the knees and chest as you rotate from side to side. The movement should be smooth and continuous.

| | |
|---|---|
| reps | 5–10 each side |
| visual cue | wheel |
| emphasis | core strength |

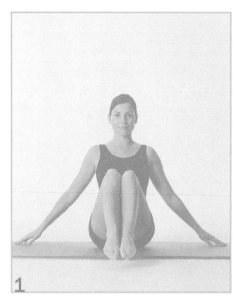

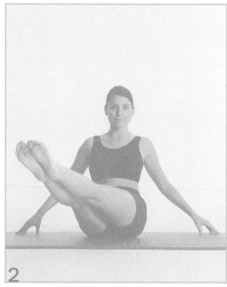

**1** Sit tall in a balanced position with your feet comfortably close to your bottom. Your hands should be out to the sides in a balancing position, and feet and hands should only lightly touch the floor.

**2** As you breathe out, lift up your legs straight in front of you, then swing your hips to the right; as you breathe in, swing back to the centre. On the next outbreath, swing to the left, and continue from side to side.

## modification

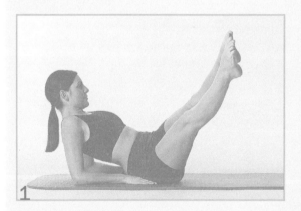

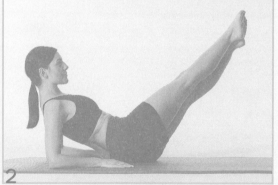

**1** To decrease the difficulty, rest on your elbows, lifting your chest to the ceiling, and try to maintain neutral. Bend your knees as you breathe in, and breathe out as you lengthen your legs.

**2** Swing your legs around to the side, holding your position at the top of the movement. Repeat to the other side.

# side kick

if you feel tension in your neck, you may wish to put a towel under your head to relieve it. The closer your supporting hand is to your body, the more challenging the position, so begin with the hand slightly further away, but not so the top shoulder rolls off the bottom shoulder.

| reps | 5–10 times each side |
| --- | --- |
| visual cue | drawn bow |
| emphasis | leg and bottom strength |

1 Lying on your right side, lengthen your legs out, making sure that your heels are in line with your hips (if your feet are behind your hipline, you may feel discomfort in the lower back). Stack your shoulders, hips, knees, and feet on top of each other. Relax your head onto your lengthened right arm, and draw your right waistline away from the floor to help you maintain a neutral position of the spine and pelvis. Place your left hand on the floor just in front of you, and draw your shoulders back and down.

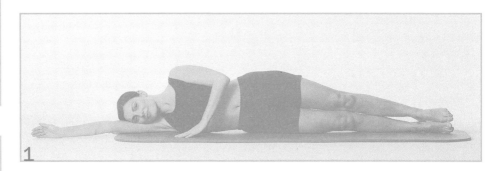

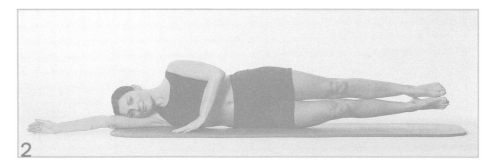

2 As you breathe out, lengthen your legs away from you as if you were reaching towards the opposite wall. As you continue to lengthen, float your legs a few inches off the floor, while maintaining a controlled and balanced position.

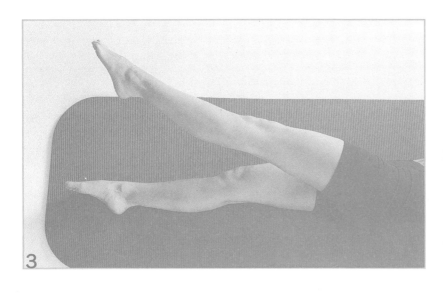

3 If you would like to challenge yourself further, slide the left leg forwards on your next outbreath in a slow kicking motion. The move should be controlled and should last for the duration of your outbreath. As you breathe in, return the top leg directly back over the bottom leg, not allowing the top leg to go behind the bottom leg. Repeat 5–10 times, then change sides. Try to keep your hand off the floor during the movement.

# side scissors

Focus on lengthening throughout this move. As you lift your legs, ensure that they don't drop back behind your hips as this will cause stress on the lower back. Bring your feet slightly forwards without moving them into a banana shape.

**! CAUTION**

**Avoid lifting your legs any higher than your hipline.**

| reps | 5–10 times each side |
|------|---------------------|
| visual cue | scissors |
| emphasis | leg and bottom strength |

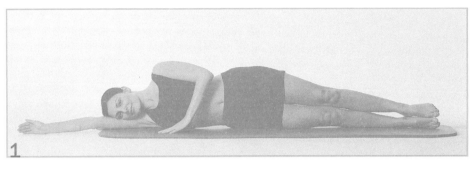

**1** Lying on your right side, lengthen your legs out, making sure that your heels are in line with your hips (if your feet are behind your hipline, you may feel discomfort in the lower back). Stack your shoulders, hips, knees, and feet on top of each other. Relax your head onto your lengthened right arm, and draw your right waistline away from the floor to help you maintain a neutral position of the spine and pelvis. Place your left hand on the floor just in front of you, and draw your shoulders back and down.

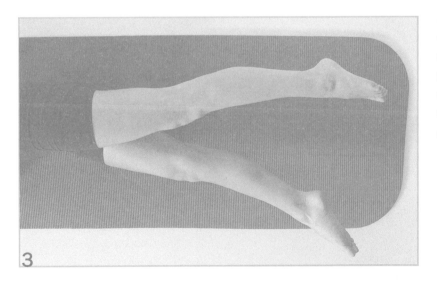

**2** As you breathe out, lengthen your legs away from you as if you were reaching towards the opposite wall. As you continue to lengthen, float your legs a few inches off the floor, while maintaining a controlled and balanced position.

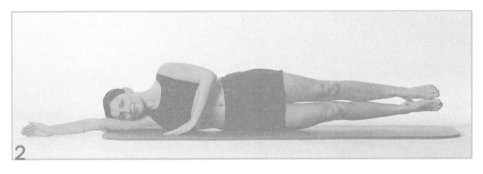

**3** As you breathe out, slide the bottom leg forwards and the top leg slightly back. As you breathe in, slide the legs the opposite way, creating a scissor action. Keep both feet off the floor and the spine and pelvis in neutral.

# side lifts

Progress through these moves over a period of sessions. Doing them all in one session will exhaust the areas of your body being worked.

**! CAUTION**

**Allow your body to lift itself to a position where it is challenged, but is not straining.**

| | |
|---|---|
| reps | 5–10 times each side |
| visual cue | rocking |
| emphasis | leg and bottom strength |

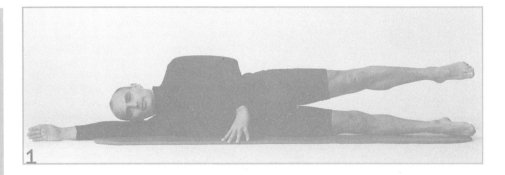

1 Lying on your right side, lengthen your legs out, making sure that your heels are in line with your hips (if your feet are behind your hipline, you may feel discomfort in the lower back). Stack your shoulders, hips, knees, and feet on top of each other. Relax your head onto your lengthened right arm, and draw your right waistline away from the floor to help you maintain a neutral position of the spine and pelvis. Place your left hand on the floor just in front of you, and draw your shoulders back and down.

As you breathe out, lift the top leg. Then, as you breathe in, lower the leg within an inch of the bottom leg, before raising it again on the next outbreath.

To advance these moves, try to lift both legs on the outbreath and lower them on the

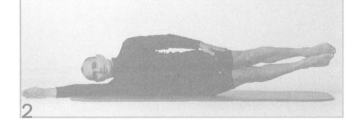

inbreath. Keep the legs within an few inches of the floor until you have completed the sequence. Then lower the legs to the floor.

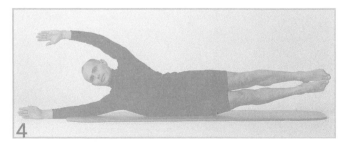

2 As a further challenge, take the front hand off the floor and stretch your arm along your side.

3 Once you have mastered these moves, try lifting the upper body on the outbreath at the same time as lifting the lower body. For extra stability, place the top hand in front of you.

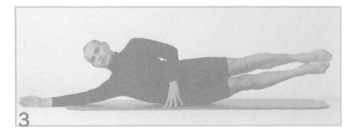

4 Now try to lift your upper body and lower body, lengthening the top arm over your head on the outbreath. As you breathe in, lower the head back to the bottom arm, the top arm back to your side, and the legs about an inch off the floor.

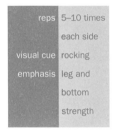

# hip rolls

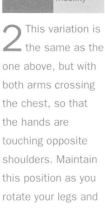
The movement should be continuous, but pause briefly in the centre before rotating in the opposite direction. Allow the rate of your breathing to control the speed of the movement.

| | |
|---|---|
| reps | 5–10 times each side |
| visual cue | child rolling |
| emphasis | waist strength and spine mobility |

1 Begin by lying on your back with your knees bent, your feet flat, and your arms open in a crucifix position. Draw your shoulders back and down, and rotate your head to the left, in a position where there is no tension in the neck. Keep your legs bent and your knees together as you breathe out, and slowly allow the knees to roll to the right side. You don't have to touch the floor with your knees, but rather rotate to a position where the knees can stay together and where there is no tension or pinching in the lower spine. As you breathe in, bring the head and legs back to the centre position. On the next outbreath, rotate the head and legs in the opposite direction.

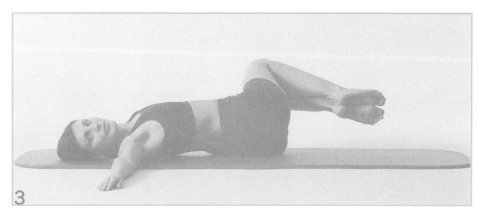

2 This variation is the same as the one above, but with both arms crossing the chest, so that the hands are touching opposite shoulders. Maintain this position as you rotate your legs and head in opposite directions.

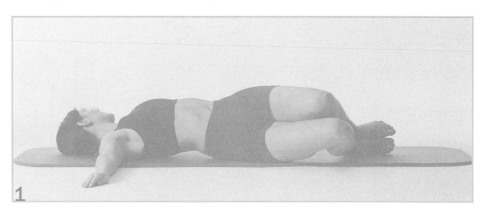

3 Once you have mastered the two positions above, try this more challenging version. Lift your feet off the floor, keeping the feet and knees together, and rotate your legs to one side as you turn your head to the other.

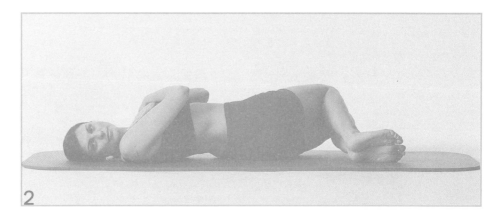

# knee circles

Imagine that you are stirring porridge with your knees, keeping the circular stirring movement of both knees the same.

**! CAUTION**

**If your lower back feels uncomfortable, return to the one-leg circle exercise.**

| | |
|---|---|
| reps | 5–10 times each way |
| visual cue | circle in air |
| emphasis | hip mobility |

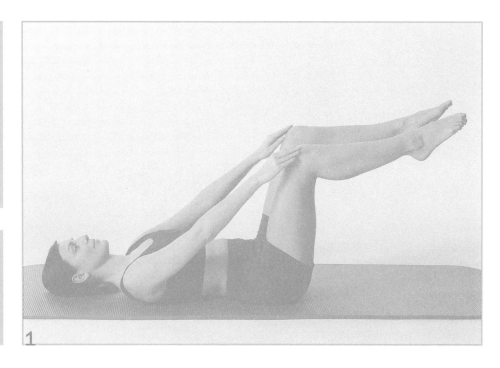

1

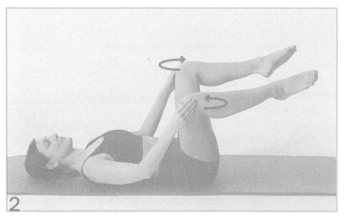

2

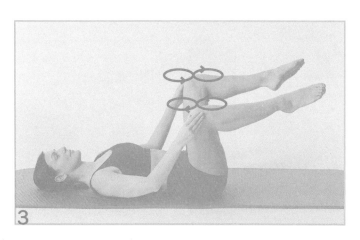

3

1 Lying on your back, lift the right leg to form a right angle, imprint the lower spine, and then lift the left leg (see the hundred on pages 52–3). Draw your shoulders back and down, and place you hands lightly on your knees. If you feel that you are unable to maintain neutral, and the lower back is increasing in size or the lower abdominals are doming, then lower one leg followed by the other. This is an advanced progression of the one-leg circle, and it will need time and practice to achieve.

2 Circle both knees in opposite directions: as you breathe out, the knees circle out and away from the centre; as you breathe in, the knees come back in towards the centre. The movement should start quite small, so imagine drawing a circle on the ceiling about the size of a small plum. Keep the feet and knees in line.

3 Once you have mastered the above moves, a more advanced version is to draw circles with your knees in opposite directions, following a figure-of-eight shape.

# the seal

As you roll, imagine that you are a ball. When you return to a balanced position, try to lengthen yourself. Always bring your pelvis back to a neutral position before rolling back again.

| | |
|---|---|
| reps | 5–10 times |
| visual cue | rolling ball |
| emphasis | abdominal strength |

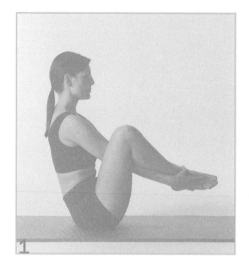

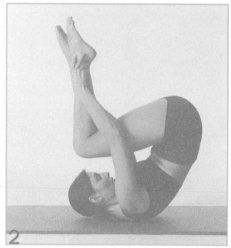

1 Sit on the floor in a balanced position, place your arms through the centre of your legs, and hold on to the outside of your feet. Draw the feet in comfortably close to your bottom and lengthen your spine as much as you can.

2 Breathe in as you roll back onto your shoulder blades: stay in a tight ball as you roll in a smooth and continuous movement. Focus on imprinting each vertebra into the mat as you roll. Breathe out as you return to a balanced position. Sit tall, and gently open and close the feet in a tapping movement three times. Breathe in, and start the roll again.

# the crab

Keep the shape tight, and roll onto your shoulder blades rather than your head.

**! CAUTION**

**Try not to throw yourself forwards as you come up, or you may risk falling forwards on your forehead.**

| | |
|---|---|
| reps | 5–10 times |
| visual cue | crab |
| emphasis | abdominal strength |

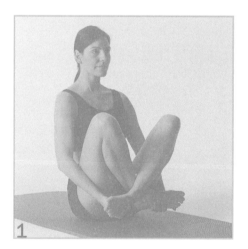

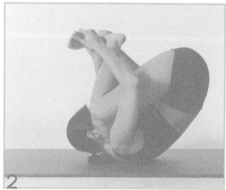

2 Breathe in as you roll back in a tight ball onto your shoulder blades. Focus on imprinting each vertebra into the mat as you roll. Breathe out as you return to a balanced position. Sit up tall, breathe in, and begin to roll once again.

1 Sit in a balanced position, cross your ankles, and reach round to take hold of your feet. Keep your feet close to your bottom, lengthen your spine, and sit up tall.

# runner stretch

To increase the stretch, move the front leg a little further forwards, then lean further into the movement.

**! CAUTION**

**Practise this move in front of a mirror to ensure that the knee and foot stay in line. If your weight pushes forwards over the front knee, this can cause discomfort to the knee joint.**

| reps | hold for 5–10 breaths |
|---|---|
| visual cue | straddling |
| emphasis | stretch |

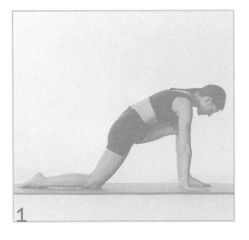

1 From a kneeling position, take a lunge forwards with your left leg until your knee and foot are in line: you should feel the stretch in the groin of your right leg. If you don't feel it, slide the left leg further back until you do. Place your hands either side of the left foot with the left toe facing forwards.

2 As you breathe out, lengthen the upper body so that you lengthen the spine into a neutral position. Place the hands on the left leg, just above the knee joint.

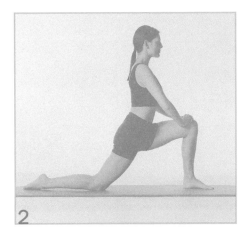

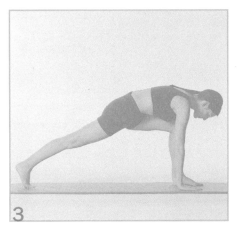

3 In order to advance the stretch, float the right knee off the floor on your next outbreath, and place your hands next to your left foot to stabilize you. Check that the front knee and ankle are in line.

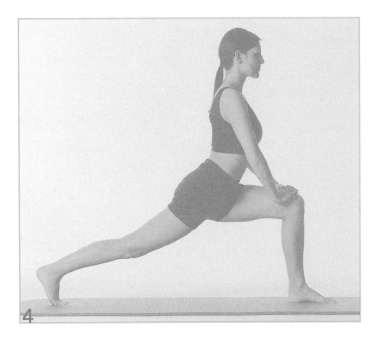

4 On your next outbreath, lengthen the upper body so that you extend the spine into a tall, neutral position, and place the hands on the front leg, just above the knee joint. Repeat on the other side. Hold the stretch each side for 15–30 seconds, then try to increase this time as you become familiar with the movement.

# up a tree

Try to keep the knees as straight as possible without locking the knee joint. This will ensure that the stretch also runs up through the back of the knee.

| | |
|---|---|
| reps | 5–10 times each side |
| visual cue | climbing |
| emphasis | abdominal strength |

**1** Lie on your back with your legs straight, and find the neutral spine postion. On your next outbreath, raise your right leg towards the ceiling and place your hands on the back of your right thigh. Try to keep your leg as straight as possible, without locking your knee. Keep your shoulders drawn back and down and your neck relaxed.

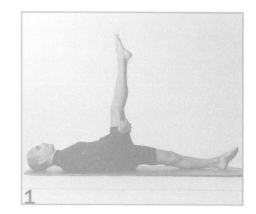

**2** On the next outbreath, start to walk your hands one over the other as you climb towards your foot: your head and shoulders will lift off the floor as you proceed. Imagine that you are climbing up a tree, walking your hands up your leg.

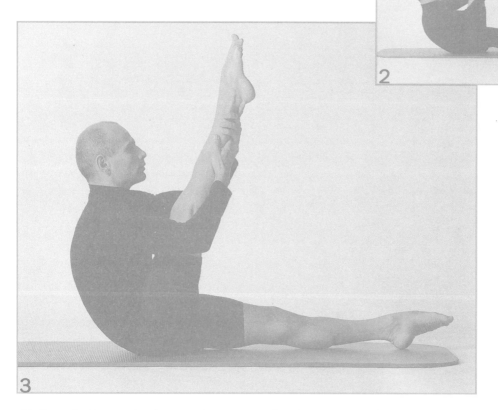

**3** Keep climbing your hands up your leg until you have gone as far as possible without overstraining. Take a breath in and as you breathe out, reverse the whole exercise walking your hands down until your head and shoulders are back on the floor.

# rocker

If your hamstrings are tight, you may find it difficult to keep the legs straight, so begin with the knees slightly bent or alternatively start with the seal and crab moves (see page 68).

**! CAUTION**

**Don't force the move as you come up, otherwise you may fall forwards.**

| | |
|---|---|
| reps | 5–10 times |
| visual cue | rocking chair |
| emphasis | abdominal strength |

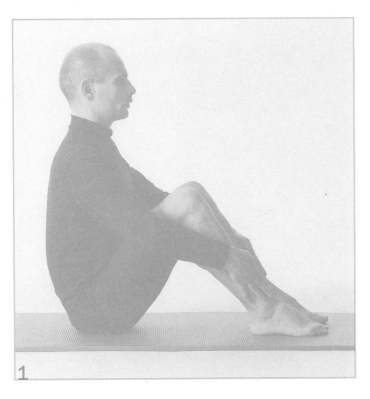

1 Sit tall with your feet comfortably close to your bottom. Place your hands on the outside of your legs, as close to your feet as possible.

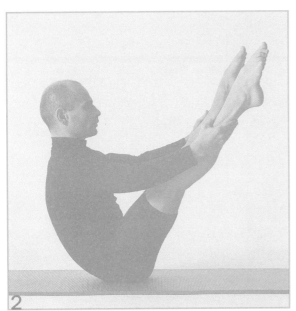

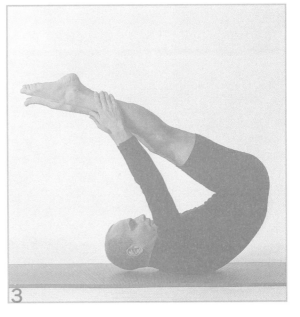

2 As you breathe out, lengthen one leg towards the ceiling. Maintaining a stable and balanced position, lengthen the other leg towards the ceiling, keeping hold of the outside of each leg just below the knee.

3 As you breathe in, begin to roll back onto your shoulders, keeping the distance between your thighs and chest the same and continuing to clasp your calves. On the outbreath, return to a balanced position, fold the legs back down, then begin the move once again.

# standing chest stretch

This exercise is aimed at stretching the major muscles of the chest called the pectorals. Stand tall in a neutral position, and think about lengthening up and through the chest and the ribcage.

| reps | 5–10 breaths |
|---|---|
| visual cue | on parade |
| emphasis | stretch |

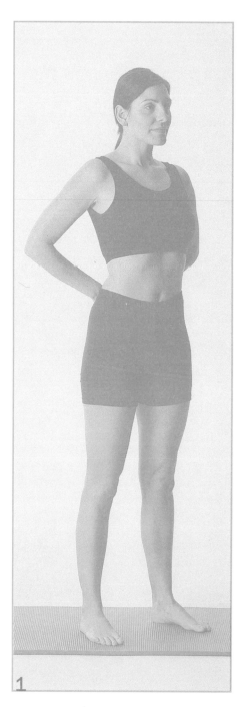

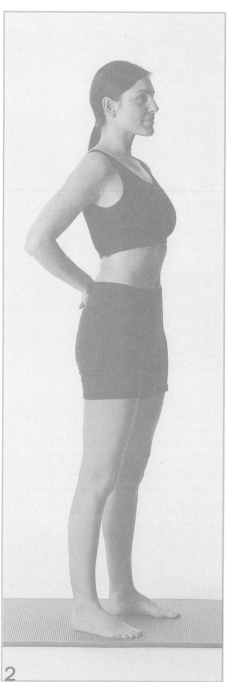

**1** Stand tall in a neutral position with your feet hip-width apart. Place your palms on your lower back with your hands comfortably close to each other. Concentrate on maintaining a neutral position and not forcing the lower back out of neutral.

**2** As you breathe out, try to draw the elbows closer together. As you do this, open the chest, stand tall, and keep your eyes looking forwards and slightly lifted as if looking over the horizon.

# chest stretch with ball

If you don't have a
ball, you can use
a chair instead.

**! CAUTION**

**Don't lock your
elbows – keep them
soft. Never force
a stretch.**

| | |
|---|---|
| reps | 5–10 |
| | breaths |
| visual cue | bowing on |
| | knees |
| emphasis | chest |

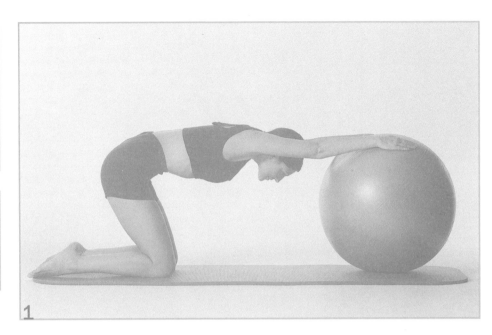

1 Kneel in front of the ball. Place your hands onto the ball, shoulder-width apart. Try not to have the ball too far away, otherwise it will feel unstable. As you breathe out, keep your hands on the ball, and sit your bottom back towards your heels. Your bottom doesn't need to touch your heels – just sit back far enough to feel a stretch through your chest muscles.

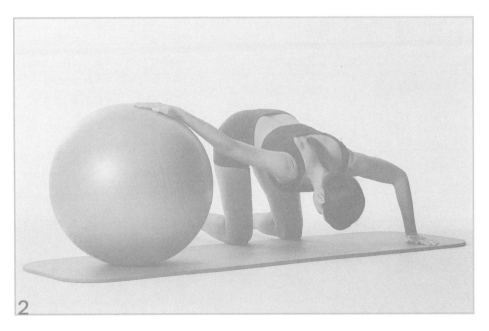

2 To stretch the upper part of your chest, kneel side-on to the ball. Take your right hand out slightly wider than your shoulder, and put the left hand onto the ball. Breathing out, gently drop the left shoulder towards the floor. As you do this, try not to rotate from the hips, just the left shoulder.

# hamstring stretch with dynaband

You can use a towel if you don't have a dynaband.

**! CAUTION**

**Don't lock the knees and don't force the stretch.**

| | |
|---|---|
| reps | 5–10 breaths each leg |
| visual cue | glass balanced on foot |
| emphasis | back of thigh |

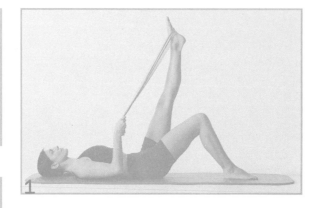

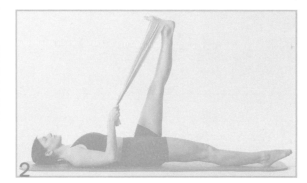

1 Lie on your back, knees bent and feet flat. Bring your right foot up towards, you and wrap the dynaband under it. Take a firm hold of the band with both hands, and as you breathe out, lengthen your right leg towards the ceiling. Keeping your leg straight and your elbows tucked in, pull gently on the band to draw your leg closer to your chest. Concentrate on maintaining a neutral spine as you do this.

2 To challenge yourself further, as you breathe out lengthen your left leg along the floor. Again, concentrate on maintaining a neutral spine.

# quad stretch

Pull the leg gently back – don't force the knee.

**! CAUTION**

**If you feel any pain in your knee, stop at once.**

| | |
|---|---|
| reps | 5–10 breaths |
| visual cue | hopscotch |
| emphasis | front of thigh |

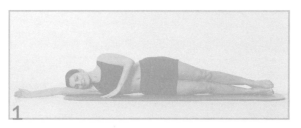

1 Lie in a side line position, maintaining a neutral spine.

2 Reach out with your right hand to take hold of your right foot, keeping your hips and knees stacked on top of each other. Gently push your foot into your hand. Add a little resistance to this move by using your hand to draw your foot closer to your bottom. You should feel the stretch in the front of your thigh as you do this.

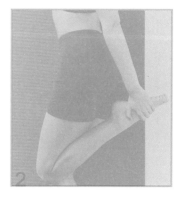

# stretch against a wall

**! CAUTION**

Don't lock your elbows, and make sure that the surface you are leaning against is strong.

| | |
|---|---|
| reps | 5 breaths each arm |
| visual cue | hand glued to wall |
| emphasis | top of chest |

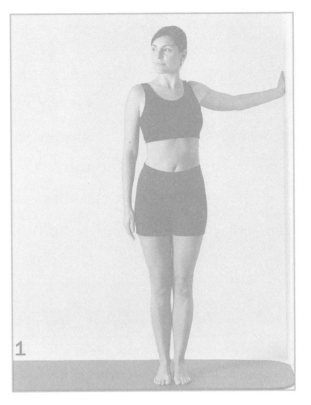

1 Stand side-on to the wall. Place your right hand on the wall, then take a small step forward with both feet. Maintain neutral spine, but with your feet close together. As you breathe out, lean slightly forwards. Hold the stretch for a few seconds, then release the stretch. Repeat 3–5 times.

# foot stretch

It's best if you do this move with your shoes and socks off.

**! CAUTION**

Make sure that the surface you are leaning against is strong.

| | |
|---|---|
| reps | 5–10 breaths each leg |
| visual cue | pushing a car |
| emphasis | stretching shin |

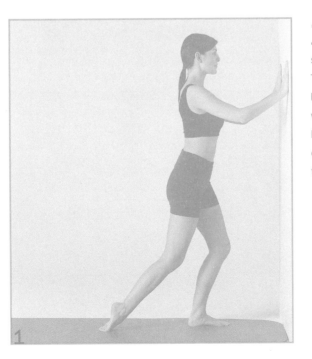

1 Stand facing close to a wall. Bend your left knee and step back with the right foot. Tuck the right toes under as you breathe out, then press into the wall lightly and bend the right knee a little further. Push down on the top of the foot to stretch this area.

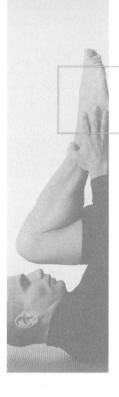

# progressions

As you progress with the Pilates technique, you can join up the individual moves to form a flowing sequence – so, instead of repeating one move 10 times, you can take, say, three moves and link them together. This "progression" enables you to increase the intensity of your workout by making it last longer, rather than by choosing more challenging moves.

## roll-up–seated spine twist–rolling back

For more details of the first and last moves see pages: 50 and 47.

Repeat these three moves as one continuous move.

| | |
|---|---|
| reps | 5–10 times |
| emphasis | control and strength |

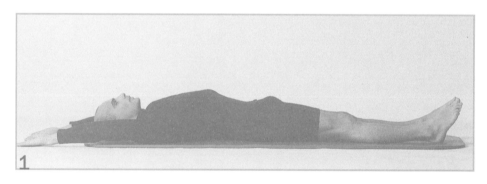

1

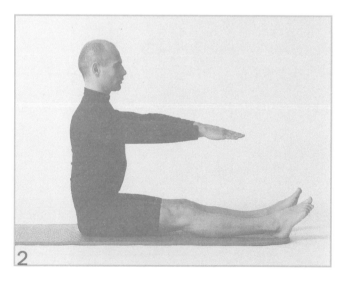

2

**1** Lie on the floor on your back with your legs straight and your arms stretched over your head. Draw your shoulders back and down.

**2** As you breathe out, begin to peel your heads and shoulders off the floor, and slowly lift your arms to the ceiling as you start to come up.

**3** As you lengthen to the top of the position, prepare to go into the seated spine twist. Put your hands together. Breathe out as you rotate to the right. Breathe in as you return to the centre. Breathe out and rotate to the left. Finally, come back to the centre with your next inbreath.

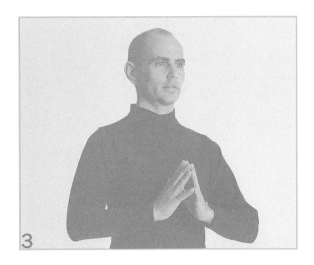

**4** On your next inbreath, roll back, coming back to a seated position on your outbreath.

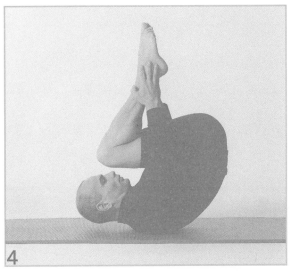

**5** Sit tall, and start again from the roll-up.

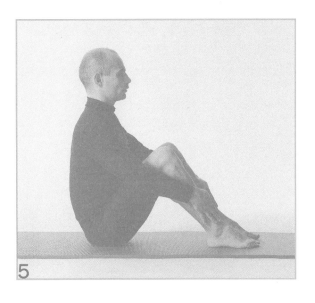

# standing spine twist–push-up–leg-pull prone

For more details of each move see the following pages: 36, 40, and 45.
The movements should flow evenly – transition from the Push up into the Leg pull prone should be smooth.

| reps | 5–10 times |
|------|------------|
| emphasis | control and strength |

PROGRESSIONS

**1** Stand tall with your hands together in a prayer position. Breathe out as you rotate to the right side, breathe in to return to the centre. Breathe out, and rotate to the left and in as you come back to the centre position.

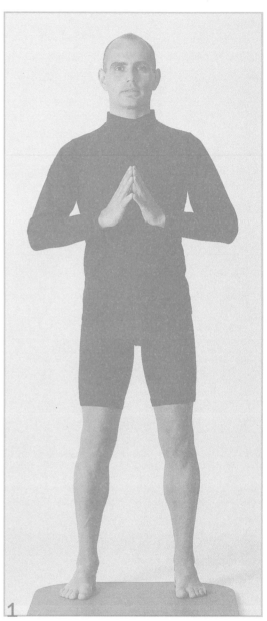

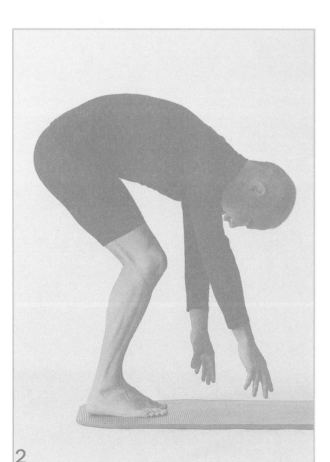

**2** Breathe out and lengthen your arms down by your side. Breathe in as you prepare to move. On the outbreath, begin the roll down.

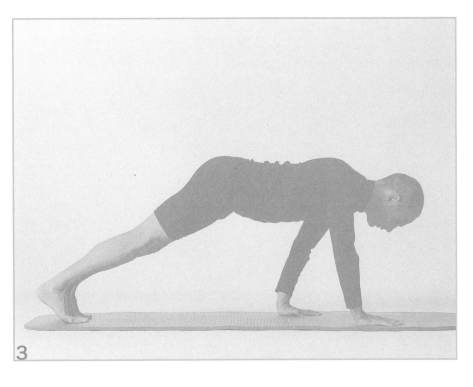

3 Choose from the modifications of the push-up position (see page 41) and perform one push.

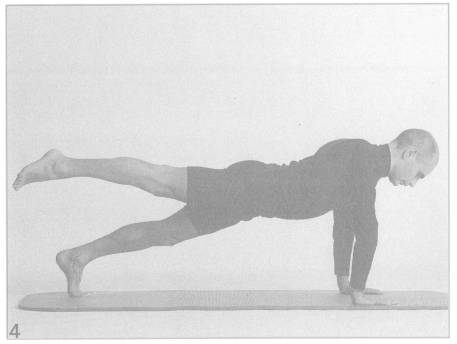

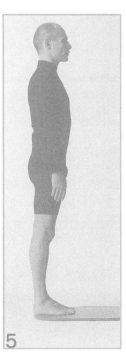

4 Set yourself in the leg pull prone – choose from the modifications on page 45. Hold this position for 5 whole breaths if possible, on the last outbreath, begin to walk the hands towards your feet. Breathe in before you begin to uncurl as you breathe out.

5 Finish in a standing neutral position. Breathe in, and begin the sequence again.

# rolling back–teaser–jackknife

For more details of
the first two moves,
see the following
pages: 47 and 51.
Try to link the
movements together.
Listen to your body.
If you become tired,
stop or lower the
level of intensity.

| reps | 5–10 times |
| --- | --- |
| emphasis | control and strength |

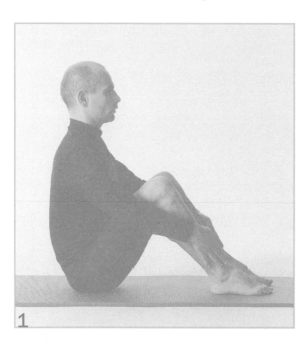

**1** Start in a seated position with your hands clasped around your ankles.

PROGRESSIONS

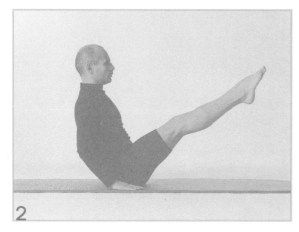

**2** As you begin to roll up out of the rolling position, hold in a balance position, and extend your legs into the teaser. Begin by using your hands beside you to find a balance position without losing neutral spine.

**3** Once you feel confident, take your hands away, and keeping them at shoulder height, reach towards your feet.

**4** As you breathe out, lengthen your chest towards your legs as if you were folding. Breathe in, then as you breathe out, open out by tilting your pelvis under.

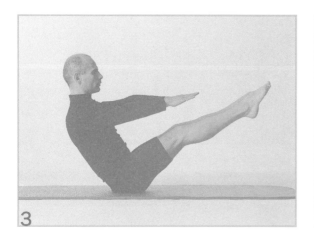

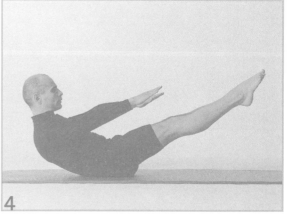

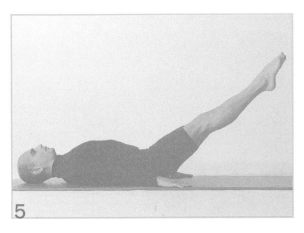

5 Slowly lower your head and shoulders to the floor whilst keeping your legs lifted in a diagonal position as you breathe out. Begin to peel the lower part of your spine off the floor.

6 As you begin to peel the spine off the floor, your legs will begin to lift over your head. Continue to peel the spine off the floor until you are resting on your shoulders and your legs are lengthened towards the ceiling.

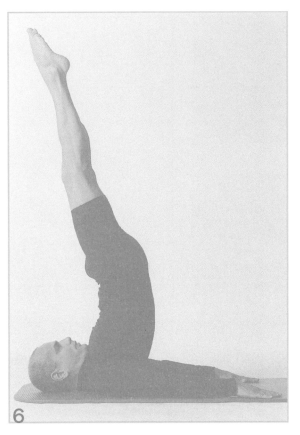

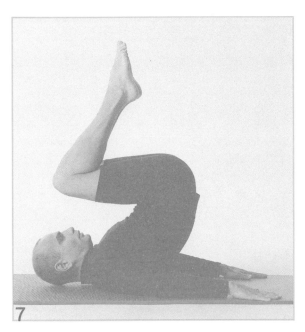

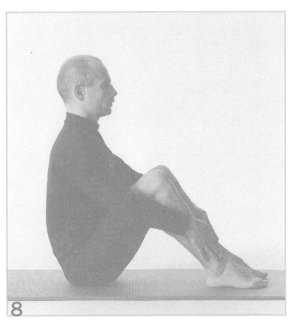

7 Hold for two breaths. On your second outbreath, draw your knees towards your chest.

8 Complete the rolling until you are sitting up in the start position.

# side bend–side kick–scissors

For more details of
each move, see the
following pages:
46, 63, and 56.
Try to link the
movements together
into a flowing
sequence.

| reps | 5–10 times |
| --- | --- |
| emphasis | strength and control |

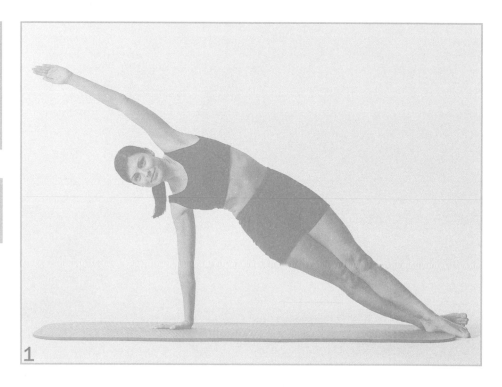

**1** Start in a side position (see page 46 for modifications). Breathe out, and lower your hips back to the floor.

## side bend modification

Rest your body on
your elbow with
the elbow directly
under your
shoulder. Bend
both knees, and
stack the knees
and feet on top of
each other.

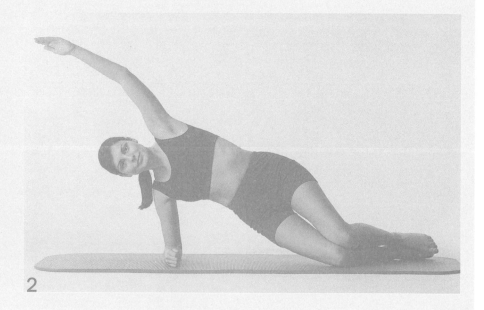

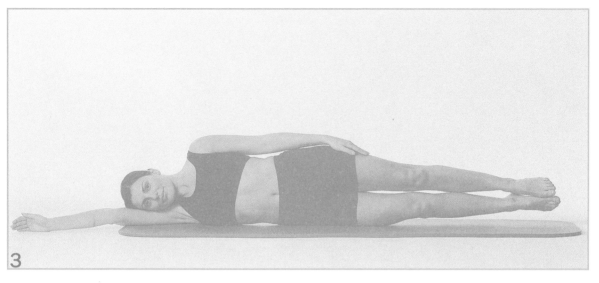

3 Slowly slide out the lower arm into the side kick position, then perform five kicks with the top leg.

4 Add on the scissor movement. As the top leg slides forward, allow the bottom leg to slide slightly back, without losing neutral spine. Beware you do not allow the lower spine to become tight and compressed. As you breathe in again, allow the top leg to slide back and the bottom leg to slide forwards. Breathe in for two slides and out for two slides. Repeat the leg slides five times in total, and complete the last set with both of your feet together.

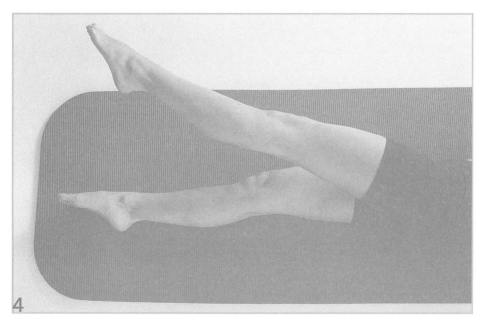

# side kick–one-leg circle

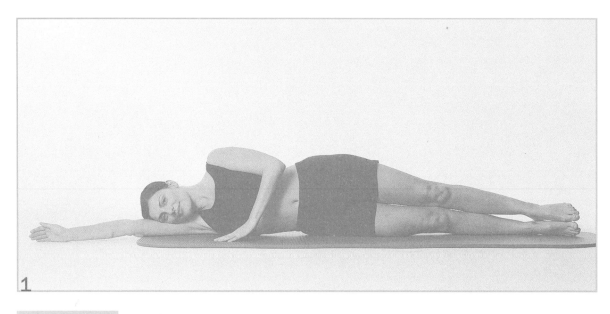

For more details of
each move see the
following pages:
63 and 55.
Try to link the
movements together
into a flowing
sequence.

| reps | 5–10 times |
| --- | --- |
| emphasis | control and strength |

1 Begin in the side line position (see page
63). Stack your shoulders, hips, knees,
and feet on top of each other. Relax your
head onto your lengthened right arm, and
draw your waistline away from the floor to
help you maintain a neutral spine and pelvis.

## advanced

2 Keeping your waistline away from the
floor, lift your legs up off the mat
together. Make sure your hips and
shoulders remain stacked.

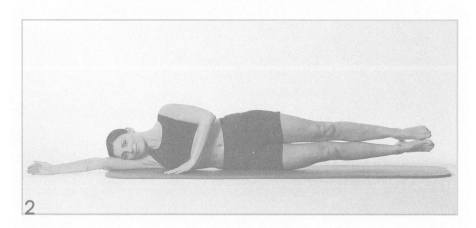

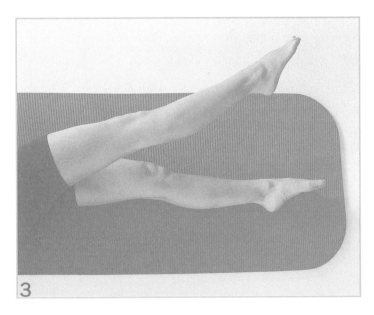

**3** Kick your top leg forward as you breathe out. Repeat this five times, and on the fifth breath, allow the leg to come back in line with the lower leg, but not to touch it. Roll over to the other side and repeat five times with the other leg. Try to make the transition as smooth as possible.

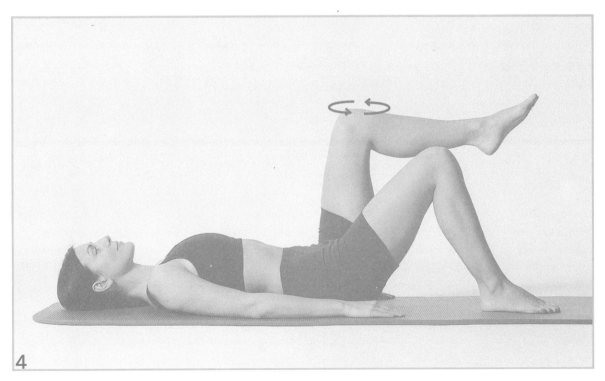

**4** Lie on your back, with knees bent and feet flat on the floor comfortably close to your bottom. Find neutral, and with your arms by your side, draw your shoulders back and down. As you breathe out, lift your left leg to form a right angle: the knee should be directly above the hip and the foot should be in line with the knee. Hold the leg in this position for five whole breaths. Focus on keeping the hips still and braced. Keeping the left knee bent, use it to draw a small circle on the ceiling. As it comes towards the centre of the body, breathe in; as it travels away, breathe out. Perform five circles in each direction, increasing the size of the circle with each one. Repeat with the other leg.

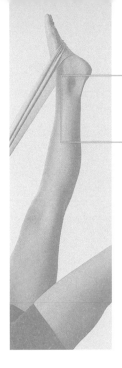

# programmes

These programmes have beginner, intermediate, and advanced levels. The levels are not based on your current fitness, but on your practice and understanding of Pilates: even if you have been training with weights or attending aerobics classes, you will still need to start with the beginner programme.

Good quality and precision are far more important than fast progression through the moves.

Modifications have also been given to allow the opportunity to make adaptations if you require, perhaps because of to your medical history or current injuries.

### Patience
Pilates most benefits those who have the greatest patience. Do not be tempted to cheat and skip ahead with the moves before you are ready. You will know when you are ready to move on by when you are able to perform the moves without losing the breathing or cheating.

### Do not rush
The slower you are able to perform the moves, the more benefits you will gain from the moves. Slow moves ensure the full use of all the muscles.

### Setting the pace
It might take a month or so to

perfect each of the levels. Do things at a pace that feels comfortable for you. If you experience any pain either during the exercise or after, stop. If pain continues, seek medical advice.

If you are sweating or shaking you are pushing yourself too hard and need to step back. As I have said before, you should expect your weaknesses to be revealed.

### Starting the programme
Initially each programme should last around an hour. You should always split your moves into two halves. In my classes, most people take around a month or so to master the exercises set out in level one. Aim to follow the programme three or four times a week if possible.

The programmes are set out in levels, but as you progress, feel free to mix and match the programmes. The programmes set out are there to give you examples of where to start.

### Don't despair
Just how fast you progress through the programmes depends on a number of factors, including how often you spend a week following the programmes, for how long, your concentration levels, your physical condition, and any other things that are happening in your lifestyle such as new job, moving home, or injuries.

Do not despair if sometimes you feel less capable of achieving movements at the higher levels than at other times. It is normal for the body to feel more tired on some days than others. Listen to what your body is telling you. A small amount of regular exercise, correctly performed, is always better than erratic overexertion. Joseph Pilates asserted that you should attempt at least 10 minutes of Pilates a day without fail. If you can only spare 10 minutes, it is best to concentrate on Rolling back (p.47) and The hundred (p. 52).

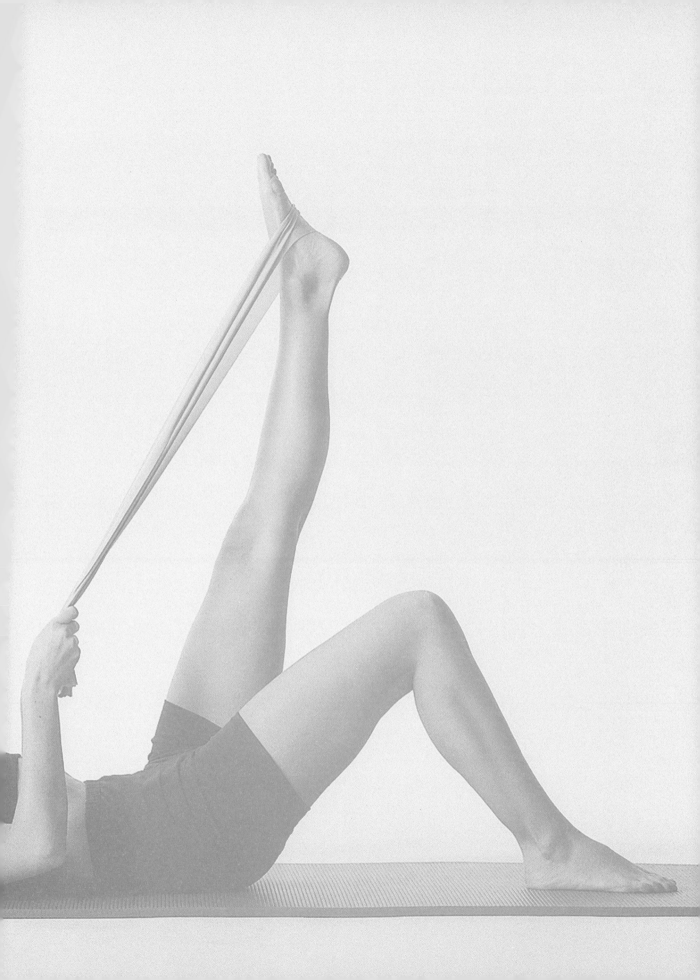

## The beginners programme

This programme has been designed to give you all
the basic tools you will need to understand the Pilates
technique. Once you have mastered the skills, move
on to the intermediate level.

| | Page | Exercise | Emphasis | Repetitions | Modification/Advance to add |
|---|---|---|---|---|---|
| | | **Warm-up** | | | |
| 1 | 22 | Breathing practice | Awareness | 1 minute | |
| 2 | 30 | Neutral spine practice | Awareness | 1 minute | |
| 3 | 37 | Spine swing | Mobility | 5–10 reps | Start with small movement range |
| 4 | 38 | Balance 1 | Balance | 5–8 breaths | Hold wall for support if needed |
| | | **Workout** | | | |
| 5 | 40 | Push-up | Strength | 5 reps | Bend knees, modify press-up position |
| 6 | 42 | Swimming | Strength | 20 reps each side | Legs only |
| 7 | 54 | Shoulder bridge | Mobility | 5–10 reps | Reduce height |
| 8 | 63 | Side kick – right side | Strength | 5–10 reps | Lower leg stays on floor |
| 9 | 52 | The hundred | Strength | 5 breaths each leg | |
| 10 | 63 | Side kick – left side | Strength | 5–10 reps | Lower leg stays on floor |
| 11 | 50 | Roll-up | Strength | 5 reps | Knees bent, begin with pelvic tilt |
| 12 | 59 | Seated spine stretch | Mobility | 5–10 reps each side | Reduce how far forward you go |
| 13 | 66 | Hip rolls | Strength/ Mobility | 5 reps each side | Feet stay on floor |
| | | **Stretch** | | | |
| 14 | 69 | Runner stretch | Stretch | 5 breaths each leg | Keep back knee on floor |
| 15 | 70 | Up a tree | Stretch/ strength | 5 times each leg | Bend knee of leg that stays on the floor |
| 16 | 72 | Standing chest stretch | Stretch | 5 breaths | |
| 17 | 74 | Quad stretch | Stretch | 5 breaths each leg | Loop towel round ankle |
| 18 | 75 | Foot stretch | Stretch | 5–10 breaths each leg | |

## The intermediate programme

Having followed the beginners programme for some time, you should have a good understanding of your neutral position, breathing, and alignment. You should also have a good understanding of your body awareness and how to stabilize the spine and pelvis.

When you are ready, you may begin the intermediate programme. Remember you can still mix in some of the beginner moves at any time. Try to keep the proramme well balanced with strength and mobility moves.

### Intermediate 1

| | Page | Exercise | Emphasis | Repetitions | Modification/Advance to add |
|---|---|---|---|---|---|
| | | **Warm-up** | | | |
| 1 | 22 | Breathing practice | Awareness | 1 minute | |
| 2 | 30 | Neutral spine Practice | Awareness | 1 minute | |
| 3 | 37 | Spine swing | Mobility | 8–10 reps | Start with small movement range |
| 4 | 38 | Balance 1 | Balance | 8–10 breaths | Hold wall for support if needed |
| | | **Workout** | | | |
| 5 | 40 | Push-up | Strength | 8 reps | Bend knees, modify press-up position |
| 6 | 42 | Swimming | Strength | 8–10 reps each leg | Arms and legs |
| 7 | 54 | Shoulder bridge | Mobility | 8–10 reps | Add arms |
| 8 | 64 | Side scissors | Strength | 8–10 reps | |
| 9 | 56 | The hundred | Strength | 5 breaths each leg x 2 | |
| 10 | 55 | One-leg circle | Mobility | 5 circles each direction | |
| 11 | 47 | Rolling back | Mobility | 5–8 reps | Hands on shins |
| 12 | 59 | Seated spine stretch | Mobility | 5–8 reps each side | Choose leg position |
| 13 | 66 | Hip Rolls | Strength/ Mobility | 5–8 reps each side | Open arms, feet off floor |
| | | **Stretch** | | | |
| 14 | 69 | Runner stretch | Stretch | 8 breaths each leg | Lift knee off the floor |
| 15 | 70 | Up a tree | Stretch/ strength | 8 times each leg | Bend knee of leg that stays on the floor |
| 16 | 72 | Standing chest stretch | Stretch | 8 breaths | |
| 17 | 74 | Quad stretch | Stretch | 8 breaths each leg | Loop towel around ankle |
| 18 | 39 | Balance 2 | Balance | 5 breaths | |

## Intermediate 2

| | Page | Exercise | Emphasis | Repetitions | Modification/Advance to add |
|---|------|----------|----------|-------------|------------------------------|
| | | **Warm-ups** | | | |
| 1 | 22 | Breathing practice | Awareness | 1 minute | |
| 2 | 30 | Neutral spine practice | Awareness | 1 minute | |
| 3 | 37 | Spine swing | Mobility | 8–10 reps | Start with small movement range |
| 4 | 38 | Balance 1 | Balance | 8–10 breaths | Hold wall for support if needed |
| | | **Workout** | | | |
| 5 | 36 | Standing spine twist | Mobility | 5–8 reps each side | |
| 6 | 44 | Plank | Strength | 5–8 breaths x 2 | |
| 7 | 54 | Shoulder bridge | Mobility | 8–10 reps | Without arms but add leg lift |
| 8 | 62 | Hip circles | Strength | 8 reps each side | Rest on elbows |
| 9 | 68 | The seal | Mobility | 8–10 reps | Rolling back (p. 47) |
| 10 | 52 | The hundred | Strength | 5 breaths each leg x 2 | |
| 11 | 57 | One-leg stretch | Strength | 5 times each leg | Lower leg that lengthens |
| 12 | 48 | Swan dive | Mobility | 8–10 reps | Choose arm positions |
| 13 | 50 | Roll-up | Strength | 8 reps | Knees bent |
| 14 | 67 | Knee circles | Mobility | 8 reps | Figure of eight |
| 15 | 46 | Side bend | Strength | 8 reps each side | Legs bent |
| 16 | 58 | Double-leg stretch | Strength/ Mobility | 8–10 reps | Arms only |
| | | **Stretch** | | | |
| 17 | 69 | Runner stretch | Stretch | 8 breaths each leg | Lengthen upper body |
| 18 | 70 | Up a tree | Stretch/ Strength | 8 times each leg | Bend other leg |
| 19 | 75 | Stretch against a wall | Stretch | 5 breaths each side | |
| 20 | 73 | Chest stretch | Stretch with ball | 5 breaths | One arm on the floor |
| 21 | 74 | Quad stretch | Stretch | 8 breaths each leg | Loop towel around ankle |
| 22 | 39 | Balance 2 | Balance | 5 breaths | |

# Intermediate 3

| | Page | Exercise | Emphasis | Repetitions | Modification/Advance to add |
|---|---|---|---|---|---|
| | | **Warm-ups** | | | |
| 1 | 22 | Breathing practice | Awareness | 1 minute | |
| 2 | 30 | Neutral spine Practice | Awareness | 1 minute | |
| 3 | 37 | Spine swing | Mobility | 8–10 reps | Start with small movement range |
| 4 | 38 | Balance 1 | Balance | 8–10 breaths | Hold wall for support if needed |
| | | **Workout** | | | |
| 5 | 52 | The hundred | Strength | 5 breaths each leg x 2 | |
| 6 | 54 | Shoulder bridge | Mobility | 10 reps | Without arms but add leg lift |
| 7 | 64 | Side scissors – right side | Strength | 10 reps | |
| 8 | 48 | Swan dive | Mobility | 10 reps | Choose arm positions |
| 9 | 64 | Side scissors – left side | Strength | 10 reps | |
| 10 | 68 | The crab | Strength/ Mobility | 10 reps | Rolling back (p. 47) |
| 11 | 66 | Hip rolls | Strength/ Mobility | 5–8 reps each side | Open arms, lift feet |
| 12 | 57 | One-leg stretch | Strength | 5 reps each leg | Lower leg that lengthens |
| 13 | 60 | The can can | Strength | 10 reps | |
| 14 | 51 | Leg-pull supine | Strength | 5 breaths x 2 | |
| 15 | 51 | Teaser | Strength | 8 reps | |
| | | **Stretch** | | | |
| 16 | 69 | Runner stretch | Stretch | 8 breaths each leg | Lengthen upper body |
| 17 | 70 | Up a tree | Stretch/ Strength | 8 times each leg | Bend other leg |
| 18 | 74 | Quad stretch | Stretch | 8 breaths each leg | Loop towel around ankle |
| 19 | 72 | Standing chest stretch | Stretch | 8 breaths | |
| 20 | 75 | Foot stretch | Stretch | 5–10 breaths each leg | |

## The advanced programme

Now your movements should be becoming more natural and fluid. This section will bring together all the moves and combine some of them into one smooth movement – these are called progressions. They become more challenging as you add in the other moves. Some of the moves are difficult, so if you find that you are struggling, return to the modifications and the intermediate programmes.

## Advanced

| | Page | Exercise | Emphasis | Repetitions | Modification/Advance to add |
|---|---|---|---|---|---|
| | | **Warm-ups** | | | |
| 1 | 22 | Breathing practice | Awareness | 1 minute | |
| 2 | 37 | Spine swing | Mobility | 8–10 reps | |
| | | **Workout** | | | |
| 3 | 40 | Push up | Strength | 8 reps | |
| 4 | 44 | Plank | Strength | 8 breaths x 2 | Add leg lifts |
| 5 | 58 | Double-leg stretch | Strength/ Mobility | 8–10 reps | Add legs |
| 6 | 80 | Rolling back– Teaser–Jackknife | Mobility/ strength | 4 reps | |
| 7 | 65 | Side lifts | Strength | 8 reps | Lift arms and legs |
| 8 | 60 | The can can | Strength | 8–10 reps | |
| 9 | 82 | Side bend–Side kick–Scissors | Strength/ Mobility | 8 reps | |
| 10 | 50 | Roll-up | Strength | 8 reps | Straighten legs |
| 11 | 52 | The hundred – both legs | Strength | 10 breaths | |
| | | **Stretch** | | | |
| 12 | 69 | Runner stretch | Stretch | 8 breaths each leg | |
| 13 | 70 | Up a tree | Stretch/ Strength | 8 times each leg | |
| 14 | 74 | Quad stretch | Stretch | 8 breaths each leg | |
| 15 | 72 | Standing chest stretch | Stretch | 8 breaths | |
| 16 | 75 | Foot stretch | Stretch | 5–10 reps each leg | |

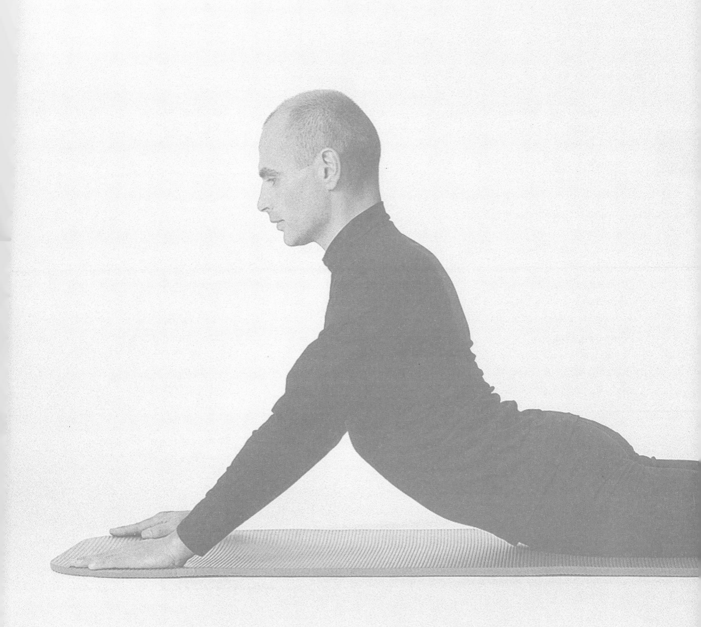

# glossary

**Abdominal muscles (abs)**: the muscles layered across the midriff that lie across each other at various angles. There are four types: the rectus abdominals, internal obliques, external obliques, and transversus abdominals.

**Aerobic exercise**: any sustained activity that works the heart and lungs, increasing the amount of oxygen in the blood.

**Alignment**: arrangement in a straight line.

**Cardiovascular**: relating to the heart or the blood vessels.

**Centering movements**: the Pilates exercises that work the centre of the body, abdominals, and back.

**Core exercises**: the Pilates movements that concentrate on strengthening the abdominal and back muscles.

**Crunching**: sit-ups where the abdominals are not engaged so much as squeezed together, shortening the space between the hips and ribcage.

**Contrology**: the name given by Joseph Pilates to his exercise method which he defined as "the science and art of coordinated body–mind–spirit development through natural movements under strict control of the will".

**C-shape**: the shape of the spine when the body is slumped over and bent due to bad posture.

**Elongation**: lengthening of the muscle. Leaner muscles develop from stretching the muscle rather than bulking it up.

**Hidden stress**: when muscle groups compensate for an injury or difficulty by using larger muscles to protect weaker ones.

**Hunching**: result of neck and shoulder tension within the trapezius muscles. Muscles here can tense up in a defensive automatic reaction.

**Hyperextension**: extending further than 180 degrees. Hyperextension occurs when the muscles tense up and the elbows or knees lock, resulting in a reverse bending.

**Imprinting**: gently pushing each vertebra into the mat, as though it were leaving an indentation.

**Lumbar curve**: the bend of the spine at the small of the back.

**Overloading**: point where the effort required by a muscle to withstand an applied weight is too great. The tissue may tear or rupture as a result.

**Powerhouse**: The name that Joseph Pilates gave to the abdominal area, found between our ribcage and hips. Pilates exercises work this area in order to create a stronger, more balanced lower back.

**Prone**: lying face downwards.

**Resistance**: an opposing force that pulls in the opposite direction to the one created by your muscle.

**Rolling**: exercises where the spine rolls over the mat, one vertebra at a time.

**Soft knees**: holding the knees relaxed and slightly bent, rather than locked.

**Supine**: lying down on the back.

**Tendon**: elastic linking tissue that connects bone to muscle.

**Tripod position**: where the feet support the body weight by distributing it evenly over three points: the ball of the foot, the middle of the heel, and the outside edge of the foot, near the little toe.

**Vertebra**: one of the bony segments that make up the spinal column.

**Visualisation**: use of mental imagery to aid the accomplishment of physical tasks – an important element of the Pilates technique that helps the mind more effectively control the body.

# index

Names of individual movements are indicated by **bold** type in the index

# acknowledgements

Many thanks to all the instructors and staff at the Pilates Institute, not only in London but also in the many other countries that continue to promote the work of Joseph Pilates through our name. This book is dedicated to our great friend and colleague Sarah Irwin, who continues to be a great inspiration to many Pilates Instructors both here in the UK and in the US where she lives.

Michael King

I hope that this book enables people to learn and utilize the Pilates technique in the same way that I have. I would like to thank Michael for his time and mentoring and to acknowledge the support received from my Mum and Dad and my boyfriend Pete.

Yolande Green